Helen Meldrum

Interpersonal Communication in Pharmaceutical Care

*Pre-publication
REVIEWS,
COMMENTARIES,
EVALUATIONS . . .*

"**T**he outstanding feature of this book is the use of a case-study approach illustrating, with real world pharmacy scenarios, the 'how to's' and 'how not to's' of not only patient counseling but also communication with co-workers. Pharmacists practicing in both community and hospital settings will invariably recall seeing themselves in these scenarios. The analysis and commentary following each case will help them self-diagnose their communication skills deficits and provide an Rx for self-treatment.

Meldrum's book doesn't avoid the issue of the difficult-to-counsel patient or co-worker conflicts but provides insights that can be applied to best meet the needs of these individuals without attempting to change their behavior."

Henry A. Palmer, PhD
*Associate Dean for Professional Affairs,
The University of Connecticut
School of Pharmacy*

"**W**ith a focus on skills-based learning, and a comprehensive collection of case studies, Helen Meldrum's *Interpersonal Communication in Pharmaceutical Care* is an excellent addition to the resources available for teaching student and practicing pharmacists. This book covers interpersonal skills in both community and hospital settings. It not only focuses on basic counseling skills, it also represents a major advance in this field by spending a great deal of time discussing the more difficult aspects, such as conflict resolution.

Meldrum offers us an interesting approach by "showing" us different ways of thinking that compel us to resist changing defensive communication styles. The bulk of this book's text consists of excellent case studies from real-life situations. These case studies not only present the spoken dialogue in an interaction, but the internal dialogue (or unspoken thoughts, as Meldrum calls them) of the various individuals is also presented. This dual approach helps us understand better the feeling component in an interaction as well as providing insight into the nature of the communication. Each case study is followed by extensive commentary. Meldrum closes the book with a discussion of new communication approaches, which will become very important with the concept of pharmaceutical care that is sweeping the profession."

Michael Montagne, RPh, PhD
Associate Professor of Social Pharmacy,
Massachusetts College of Pharmacy

"**T**his concise and very readable book combines a useful review of interpersonal communications theory with material that simulates the reality of the pharmacist's workplace, be it in the community or institutional setting.

This book would be very valuable in pharmacy practice courses, a positive reinforcer for those students going into their experiential program for the first time. The positive solutions approach to communications problems advocated and demonstrated by the author gives readers a renewed sense of confidence in their ability to deal successfully with interpersonal communication."

Ronald W. McLean, MS, RPh
Interim President and Dean,
Albany College of Pharmacy

"*Interpersonal Communication in Pharmaceutical Care* is well written and easily read. It is a wonderful collection of practical cases that routinely occur in the community and hospital setting. The practical nature of the book and the applicability to pharmacy practice will make it a must read for every communications class. The cases are a rich collection of practical and routine problems that face pharmacists every day. Students and other readers will enjoy the titles that lead into the cases that will place them instantly in the scenario. The author's insightful way of describing both the spoken and unspoken thoughts of the person in the case bring relevance and meaning to the examples. I especially appreciated how the author analyzed the communication strategy used in each case and offered practical solutions for handling the cases in several different ways. These differing strategies will serve to foster a great deal of discussion in classroom situations when the book is utilized in a teaching setting."

Kathleen A. Karnik, PharmD
Assistant Dean for Clinical Affairs,
Creighton University

"Dr. Meldrum has written a communication text that fills a gap in the currently available pharmacy literature. Her book, *Interpersonal Communication in Pharmaceutical Care*, calls upon each pharmacist and pharmacy student to evaluate his or her own skills in communication and then motivates the individual to effect a positive change in how he or she approaches the communication process. . . . Dr. Meldrum challenges the reader to take responsibility for the personal contributions brought to a conversation. She provides specific suggestions on how to begin to effect needed changes in communication skills.

I found the text a refreshing addition to available resources because it focuses on minimizing those barriers that we have the most control over—our own skills in communication. Dr. Meldrum helps empower the pharmacist to become proactive in interpersonal communication and in so doing enhance the individual's effectiveness in working with customers and co-workers."

Jana L. Jirak, PharmD
Externship Director and Associate
Professor, Ferris State University

Interpersonal Communication in Pharmaceutical Care

PHARMACEUTICAL PRODUCTS PRESS
Pharmaceutical Sciences
Mickey C. Smith, PhD
Executive Editor

New, Recent, and Forthcoming Titles:

Principles of Pharmaceutical Marketing edited by Mickey C. Smith

Pharmacy Ethics edited by Mickey C. Smith, Steven Strauss, John Baldwin, and Kelly T. Alberts

Drug-Related Problems in Geriatric Nursing Home Patients by James W. Cooper

Pharmacy and the U.S. Health Care System edited by Jack E. Fincham and Albert I. Wertheimer

Pharmaceutical Marketing: Strategy and Cases by Mickey C. Smith

International Pharmaceutical Services: The Drug Industry and Pharmacy Practice in Twenty-Three Major Countries of the World edited by Richard N. Spivey, Albert I. Wertheimer, and T. Donald Rucker

A Social History of the Minor Tranquilizers: The Quest for Small Comfort in the Age of Anxiety by Mickey C. Smith

Marketing Pharmaceutical Services: Patron Loyalty, Satisfaction, and Preferences edited by Harry A. Smith and Stephen Joel Coons

Nicotine Replacement: A Critical Evaluation edited by Ovide F. Pomerleau and Cynthia S. Pomerleau

The Honest Herbal: A Sensible Guide to the Use of Herbs and Related Remedies, Third Edition by Varro E. Tyler

Herbs of Choice: The Therapeutic Use of Phytomedicinals by Varro E. Tyler

Interpersonal Communication in Pharmaceutical Care by Helen Meldrum

Interpersonal Communication in Pharmaceutical Care

Helen Meldrum

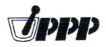

Pharmaceutical Products Press
An Imprint of the Haworth Press, Inc.
New York • London • Norwood (Australia)

Published by

Pharmaceutical Products Press, an imprint of The Haworth Press, Inc., 10 Alice Street, Binghamton, NY 13904-1580

The development, preparation, and publication of this work has been undertaken with great care. However, the publisher, employees, editors, and agents of The Haworth Press are not responsible for any errors contained herein or for consequences that may ensue from use of materials or information contained in this work. The opinions expressed by the author(s) are not necessarily those of The Haworth Press, Inc.

Library of Congress Cataloging-in-Publication Data

Meldrum, Helen.
    Interpersonal communication in pharmaceutical care / Helen Meldrum.
        p.   cm.
    Includes bibliographical references and index.
    ISBN 1-56024-867-X (alk paper).
    1. Communication in pharmacy. I. Title.
    [DNLM: 1. Interpersonal Relations. 2. Communication. 3. Pharmaceutical Services. QV 737
M518i 1994]
RS56.M45   1994
615.5'8'014–dc20   93-31220
                                                                                            CIP

CONTENTS

ABOUT THE AUTHOR

Helen Meldrum is Associate Professor of Psychology and Communication at Massachusetts College of Pharmacy and Allied Health. She has been teaching interpersonal skills to pharmacy students and practitioners since the early 1980s and has lectured and consulted to Northeastern and U.R.I. Colleges of Pharmacy, as well as with continuing education programs throughout the country. Before moving to M.C.P.A.H.S., Helen was the Director of Communication Studies as well as the Director of Education and Student Assessment at Bradford College in Bradford, Massachusetts. As principal partner in Communication Counseling Associates of Somerville, Massachusetts, she has consulted to numerous HMOs, hospitals, and retail pharmacy associations. Dr. Meldrum earned an undergraduate degree in communication education at Emerson College, a master's degree in consulting and counseling psychology at Harvard and a doctorate in psychology and education at Clark University.

Foreword

I was delighted to be invited to write the foreword for Dr. Meldrum's book, *Interpersonal Communication in Pharmaceutical Care*. Over the past several years, it has become more and more evident that the key role for pharmacists, no matter what their practice specialty or site, is their ability to counsel and interact with patients in a manner that enhances their drug therapy outcomes. Pharmacists have more contact with patients than any other health care practitioners and they are the most available, therefore interpersonal skills are essential in order for them to be effective practitioners. This manual provides a series of vignettes and cases that illustrate key components of the interpersonal skills that a hospital or community pharmacist must have. It is a unique text in that it is written by an insightful and skilled communications expert who also understands the intricacies of pharmacy practice and the need for pharmacist-patient counseling skills. This manual will serve as an excellent resource for pharmacy practitioners, students, and other health care practitioners as they seek to enhance their interpersonal skills.

Dick R. Gourley, PharmD
Dean, College of Pharmacy
University of Tennessee

Preface

This book would not exist if not for the contributions of my former students and workshop participants. Although it will seem hard to believe at times, all of the cases featured in this volume are based on transcripts of actual interactions between pharmacists, patients, customers, and co-workers. Participants in my interpersonal skills classes and workshops wrote the cases for the purpose of group discussion, so they have been made "public" on at least one previous occasion. The author, while serving as group facilitator, tried to encourage sensitive, thoughtful discussion of the dynamics of the cases while avoiding a pattern of blaming any one person featured in the dialogue.

At the time the cases were written by the participants, they were encouraged to change all of the names of the parties involved. The author has changed the names and identifying characteristics again to further safeguard confidentiality. Participants were informed that the cases might be rewritten for use in the instructor's other workshops or for educational publications. Care has been taken to select cases for this volume that are representational. For example, of the 800 case studies collected by the author, approximately 100 are of customers or patients expressing unhappiness over not being able to get another refill. With such an overlap of variations on the same theme, the author has taken the liberty of forming some "composite" responses that are blended in with the original case writer's reactions.

The purpose of making these case studies available is to provide an additional resource of concrete, realistic examples of interpersonal encounters in pharmacy practice. Hopefully, the material in this text will provide further illustration of the more theoretically based books and journal articles currently available. There is no attempt herein to offer another text providing extensive theoretical and conceptual information about communication models and re-

search. The case studies and the commentary that follows each
scenario form the heart of this volume. The debriefing section following each case study is not meant to be exhaustive or definitive.
There are more insights to be derived from each case and the readers
are invited to look for them. Also, much of the advice offered for
how to handle "difficult people" is not expected to be relevant if the
problem person is chemically or mentally impaired.

Some readers may feel that this book is overly demanding in its
expectations of the pharmacist's behavior. In an ideal world, there
would be workshops to help patients and customers to communicate
effectively with their pharmacists and other health care providers.
This is the burden of having expertise and professionalism in human
relationships. We cannot do anything about the behavior of our
customers and patients; we can only model a better way of interacting. This volume is lacking a balance of case studies that portray
very rewarding situations for the pharmacist. Perhaps that is because
the practitioners who attend the author's workshops often come
trying to get help with problematic situations. Readers are invited to
contact the author to offer additional case studies that highlight the
more positive encounters that happen every day in pharmacy practice.

Acknowledgements

So many people have been helpful in the production of this text. Laura Puzniak and Karen Mutch-Jones have borne the largest share of the production and editorial tasks. Dr. Bill Rando, my lifelong learning partner and colleague has influenced my "frame" on human behavior for over two decades now and I know we will continue to share our significant learning together. Pam Jack Polhemus has taught me much about the spirit of a writer and the importance of doing my life's work. I owe thanks to E. J. Koch for enlightening me about the dark side of interpersonal behavior. The learning community of Bradford College and its students, colleagues, and administrators were consistently supportive. Family like my mother and father, Brian, Beth, and others have offered much encouragement. Dr. Mickey Smith, who reminds me that "books are never really finished, only abandoned," is thanked for his infinite patience and faith.

Again, my greatest debt is to my students and workshop participants who have taught me about the human condition and what is possible.

Helen Meldrum
Somerville, MA

Chapter 1

Essential Interpersonal Skills for Pharmacy Practice: Communication in Counseling and Conflict Contexts

Effective interpersonal communication may be the most important professional and personal skill that we can develop. Every facet of our lives is affected by our ability or inability to relate with others. And yet, "People do not develop interpersonal competence by understanding theory" (Glasser, 1983, p. 1). If this is the case, why write yet another book on interpersonal communication? Many other authors have dedicated themselves to this very task with greater and lesser degrees of success. In fact, by the 1970s, researchers had identified 126 different operational definitions of communication in the published texts available that address this topic (Dance and Larson, 1972). This book will not belabor the debate over the conceptual components of what constitutes interpersonal communication. Instead, the text will focus on actual examples and illustrations of communication efforts in pharmacy settings. But before we move on to an intensive examination of each case study, it makes sense to at least "foreshadow" the essential skills that are necessary in pharmacy counseling and conflict management situations. Further, we will examine why it is so difficult to consistently achieve effective communication.

Interpersonal skills can be studied most simply by looking at basic message sending and receiving skills. Obviously, these messages can be either verbal or nonverbal and are invariably a mixture of both. For the purposes of providing a vocabulary to analyze the case studies to come, the discussion in this chapter will focus on how *verbal* sending and receiving skills can be improved. In particular, we will examine personal communication barriers, effective questioning, taking ownership in language use, being specific, assertion skills, conflict management, listening, and empathic counseling techniques. Finally, we will review why it is so difficult to improve these important skills.

PERSONAL BARRIERS TO COMMUNICATION

The world of pharmacy has no shortage of barriers to optimal professional practice. At a recent workshop, the author and the pharmacy audience generated a list of over 20 factors that impede success. Lack of time and pressure to fill scripts seems to loom largest in people's minds, and there is no denying the reality that even after mandatory counseling became effective nationwide, there are still not enough pharmacists to fill the consultative role. Some pharmacies have yet to be redesigned to meet this challenge, and on a recent visit to a Veterans Administration hospital, the author commented to the Pharmacy Director about the bulletproof three-inch glass separating the patients and the pharmacists. As if this weren't bad enough, the microphone system used to talk through the window had been broken for months, which left only the options of shouting and lip reading. So much for privacy. (Still, by the time this book is published, major redesigns will have taken place.)

Of course, there are the barriers arising from the patient as well. Even if patients have an excellent command of the language (which is not always the case), they are often in an angry state because the pharmacy is in essence the "last stop" on a "wasted" day that began with a medical receptionist, moved on to a nurse practitioner, and, after more waiting, to the physician, then to the lab tech, back to a practitioner, and checking out with the insurance clerk before advancing to the last "dumping grounds": the pharmacy.

The hard facts of the matter are that pharmacists cannot always immediately do something to completely remove the barriers constructed by the patient or those inherent in the environment. However, the pharmacists *can* always minimize the barriers and

time & pressure

keep from making the situation worse. Developing the ability to act instead of simply react is key. The pharmacists' own psychological mind-set generates a frame of reference that is used as a yardstick to measure and evaluate the behavior of customers, patients, and colleagues. We are constantly tempted to shift the blame for poor communication over to the other party when it's only ourselves that we have any control over. The case studies that follow in the next chapters illustrate over and over again that the pharmacists have all the information needed to improve the situation right in their heads (see "Unspoken Thoughts" in cases to come). Still, the pharmacists' reaction to psychological threat from a customer or colleague is as automatic and fast as the reflex that makes us recoil when we brush up against a hot surface.

This text takes the position that human defensiveness is the number one barrier to personal effectiveness. Because we can get defensive so quickly, we have a strong perception of limited alternatives: "Well, what else was I supposed to do? The customer was such a pain in the rear that he didn't deserve any better." Sound familiar? Communicologists Deetz and Stevenson sum up the process like this: "In times of difficulty, many people spend more energy on wishing they were someone else or somewhere else or with someone else than on exploring how to make productive changes in their communication behavior" (1986, p. 3). Quite obviously, this process constitutes the proverbial waste of energy and leads to severe burnout in a short period of time.

Another barrier in pharmacy practice is the assumption that as pharmacists we communicate as well as we need to (Habel, 1991). We "get by" with only the occasional interpersonal scrape. So why change when it requires such hard work and effort? Instead, it is easier to distort our level of competence and rationalize that if it was good enough for our preceptors and extern supervisors then it's good enough for us. However professional our role models were, it is not reasonable to assume that we learned all that there is to be learned from them. The pharmacy student socialization process is not a comprehensive one, because if it were, we would all have a better sense of accurate self-diagnosis for what skills need improvement. An effective barrier to change is the unconscious belief that our preceptors were good role models and that we learned perfectly from them. In fact, just the opposite is sometimes true. I once had a pharmacy student tell me that her preceptor passed along some wisdom that sounded like this: "Watch how I get rid of this old bag!"   ↤ attribution

It is clear how easy it is to frame the situation so that the customer or the co-worker is the one to blame. A common defensive reaction is to blurt out "You're not listening," rather than cross-examine ourselves about how we might not have been as clear as possible. True, at times the other party *is* contributing negatively to the interaction. Still, more than simply being "nice" to them, or perhaps browbeating ourselves for "losing it," we should focus on what we can do "even better" next time (that is, if we get a second chance). This discussion is not meant as a negative commentary on the many hard-working pharmacists who are trying their best, but rather a reminder of how easy it is to assume that we are well-equipped for all our present and future communication needs. Inaccurate assumptions about our communication abilities keep us from developing the motivation to do the hard work of change (Habel, 1991).

If a pharmacist is "stuck" behind his or her own personal barriers what might that sound or look like? Although the reader will see many examples of these phenomena in the cases to come, it seems useful to examine some typical statements of resistance to changing automatic, defensive communication responses (Nelson-Jones, 1990):

Passive Thinking: "Until she stops being that way to me, I'm not going to deal with her at all." What this is *really* saying: "I'm not capable of making a creative first move to stop this vicious cycle we're in."

No Alternative Thinking: "I had no choice but to tell him what I thought of him very directly." What this is *really* saying: "There was nothing else in the universe or in infinity that I could have done so don't argue or give me any constructive criticism."

Excuse Me Thinking: "He made me so mad that I couldn't help swearing at him." What this is *really* saying: "I'm justified in contributing to the interpersonal violence in this world."

Attributional Thinking: "It's all your fault that this turned out like this." What this is *really* saying: "I couldn't have possibly contributed in the least little bit to our interaction."

Blind to Consequence Thinking: "If you're not prepared to be reasonable, I don't give a damn." What this is *really* saying: "I'm going to coerce you to try to get what I want; I don't anticipate you walking out."

Past-Anchored Thinking: "Because you've let me down before I find it impossible to believe you." What this is *really* saying: "Even if you've started to act differently, I'll be blind to it or I'll feel like I can't trust what I see."

Role-Fixated Thinking: "I can't say that." What this is *really* saying: "I've never said anything like that before and since it doesn't sound like me, I won't risk trying anything new even if I feel frustrated and stuck."

Fatalistic Thinking: "You can't change human nature." What this is *really* saying: "I'm not expending any effort on change and I don't expect you to . . . that's the bargain we're striking."

It is quite clear from the preceding statements that people don't often see the perceptual barriers that they erect in moments of defensiveness. Ironically, the people listening to these statements are more likely to be hearing and reacting to the second level of statements about what is *really* being said. If we could all remember how little consciousness is present in these moments of defensiveness we might be able to better appreciate that most messages are not intended to be insulting but are rather a reflection of our self-blindness to barriers.

Why so much attention to the personal barriers erected by the pharmacist? There are many other texts, journal articles, and training programs designed to help pharmacists resolve difficult barriers emanating from the patient (e.g., pharmaceutical companies often sponsor programs on communicating with special needs patients), and there are consultants who travel around the country helping pharmacy managers redesign the environmental barriers that may not allow for privacy and optimal communication. This text highlights barriers arising from the pharmacist because of the author's strong skills-based orientation focused on taking personal responsibility. We cannot always do something to change the other person or completely rearrange the circumstances of the encounter, but we can *always* do something to improve our own effectiveness. Positive change often brings feelings of relief, which lessens our tendency to feel chronically burnt out and stuck.

EFFECTIVE QUESTIONING SKILLS

Everyone asks questions, but few people ask good questions that facilitate conversation. As a consequence, if we have dinner with someone who has just come back from a year-long, round-the-world trip, and we ask only a series of closed-framed questions, we could actually experience the traveler as a boring conversationalist. As we pay the check, we might wonder why our dinner partner wasn't more interesting. In attributing dullness to our friend, we miss the role that we played in controlling the conversation. Obviously, an opportunity to learn and be entertained was lost, but no tragedy ensued. However, should we lack vital questioning skills, we can do a lot more damage when attempting to conduct a patient interview or take a medication history.

Think of the construction of questions as existing on a continuum from very highly open to totally closed and leading. Open questions let the respondent choose from a wide range of options. Closed questions only allow for a narrow range of responses and pull for simple recall of data rather than higher level synthesized thinking. Consider the following examples that might be asked of either a patient or a co-worker (Tuttle, 1985).

Very Open:

How are you feeling?
What can you tell me about your experience in pharmacy school?

Open:

How do you expect this medication will work for you?
Where do you think you'll be in ten years?

Moderately Open:

How do you feel about trying a generic?
What continuing education programs would help you to do your job better?

Moderately Closed:

From this list of practitioners, whom should I contact about your refills?
Which of the anti-depressants do you think is the most effective?

Highly Closed:

Do you prefer generic or name brand?
Do you feel you have adequate health insurance coverage?

Totally Closed and Leading:

You don't believe all that stuff in the media about generics, do you?
You can cover for me tomorrow night, right?

In terms of building relationships with co-workers or customers, it is also best to think very carefully about your use of "why" questions (Tannen, 1986). Being asked why often makes people defensive because most people cannot give rational plausible reasons for doing or not doing the things they do. For example, "Why didn't you finish your antibiotic?" implies strong criticism, which patients will no doubt hear as a needless guilt trip (they were feeling better so what's the big deal, right?). It is better to come right out with the reasons for your concern or the thoughts that are causing you to ask the questions in an effective and specific way: "Most people don't realize that it's important to finish an antibiotic round because of the way that infections can appear to be gone but actually linger and also because not finishing can leave people resistant to the reintroduction of antibiotics. Has that been the case with you? Or is there some other reason that you didn't finish that you feel you can tell me about?" Questions can be designed in such a way as to help patients and co-workers be more precise and revealing.

The U.S. Indian Health Care Service has systematized a series of questions designed to help pharmacists interact more with their patients. The idea is to use questions to get the patient to do more of the talking and the pharmacist to do less. This approach helps lessen the burnout factor for the pharmacist who inevitably gets tired of saying the same things over and over again many times a day (e.g., "Take three times a day, one-half hour before meal time"). The questions pull the focus toward what the patient already knows and leaves the pharmacist to clarify misperceptions or to fill in the gaps in the patient's understanding (Gardner, Boyce, and Herrier, 1991).

For an initial new medical consultation, the following open-ended questions are recommended:

- What did the doctor tell you the medication is for?
- How did the doctor tell you to take the medication?
- What did the doctor tell you to expect?

And to *verify* the patient's understanding:

- Just to make sure I didn't leave anything out, can you please tell me how you are going to take your medicine?

For repeated contact with patients on maintenance-type medications the program recommends:

- What do you take the medication for?
- How do you take it?
- What kind of problems are you having?

There are advantages to asking skillful questions, but we must also remember that questions are heard on both the content and emotional levels (Tannen, 1986). For example, co-worker 1: "Let's do these IVs before we work on the med cassettes." Co-worker 2: "Why?" Co-worker 1: "Okay, we don't have to." Even "good" open-ended questions are often used in our society to carry the negative weight of criticism, rather than such "undiscussables" being stated more directly. Instead of saying, "I'd like it if we could do it this way and here is why . . ." we are socialized to say, "Why are you doing it that way?" which, paradoxically, makes the receiver *even more* defensive.

Some people try to initiate relationships by asking questions and others think people should "speak up" if they have something to say. Some folks think it's important to open a conversation by talking themselves. Still others wait to be asked questions. Imagine our pharmacist waiting to be asked while our patient is waiting to be told. Of course, neither will ever really talk and, as in the earlier example of the dull dinner partner, each can blame the other for his or her dissatisfaction (Tannen, 1986). Still, two-way talk *must* happen for real learning to occur. The U.S. Department of Health and Human Services conducted a study that proved that people remember 20% of what they hear and 90% of what they themselves say (Arnold and McClure, 1989). If the pharmacist cannot facilitate an effective discussion about how the patient should take his or her medication, then the chances are that the patient will be noncompliant. In fact, a recent U.S. Inspector General's report suggests that 45% of the general population are not taking their medicines correctly. The noncompliance problem will not be resolved until pharmacists "recondition" themselves and their patients in the art of true dialogue.

TAKING OWNERSHIP IN LANGUAGE

Communicators must be able to "own" feelings and thoughts, and to take responsibility for their behavior. In owning our feelings and thoughts, we show that we accept them rather than blame others for creating them or pretend they don't exist. Using ownership language habitually shows a commitment toward being nonjudgemental toward others (Meldrum, 1986).

At any given time human beings may demonstrate one of three basic "ways of being" in the world:

OWNING: "I am mad."

BLAMING: "You make me furious."

DENIAL: "Oh no, I'm not mad."

It is easier to identify thoughts and feelings and communicate them to others when they are owned. In the blaming mode, communicators are attempting to place responsibility for negative feelings away from themselves by pinning them onto others. Denial is a refusal to acknowledge personal thoughts or intentions. The goal of effective communicators is "to own up to" messages sent and to examine them for remnants of blame or denial.

We have all been on the receiving end of blaming language. These statements are often blurted out in an evaluative and critical manner filled with explicit or implicit "shoulds," "oughts," and "don'ts." Some forms of non-ownership in language are more insidious, with responsibility often being shifted to some unknown "they": "People won't like it much if you do that," "Everyone else thinks you should. . . ." Ownership messages are confined to description. Rather than "You make me so angry," an owned statement would be: "I get angry when you come onto shift late without calling while I have made other plans but feel obligated to continue to cover for you."

If communicators in dialogue can accept that each person's responses are properties of the communication system rather than unchangeable personality traits, they can begin to identify what each contributed to the creation of the dynamic. In viewing communication difficulties from this perspective, defensiveness is reduced, options are increased, and responsibility is shared.

Ownership statements may be the most valuable when making complaints, when offering advice, when feelings have been hurt, when there is a history of difficult conflicts, when there are differences of opinion, or when there are power differences (Deetz and Stevenson, 1986). Becoming aware of our own message construction is never easy, in part because of the rapid speed of back and forth conversation. Still, as we will see in the case studies to come, it is often the presence of blaming or denial messages that creates a defensive and destructive communication climate. To give a final example, imagine the customer's response if, instead of saying (as advocated in the previous section): "Just to make sure I didn't leave anything out, can you tell me how you're going to take the medication?" the pharmacist "accidentally" said: "Just to make sure you've got this straight, can you tell me how you're going to take this medication?" Obviously, the phrasing of just a few words makes a huge difference in how the message will be perceived. Along with ownership, communicators must take care to be as specific as possible.

BEING SPECIFIC

Taking responsibility for our own behavior can be made easier by speaking concretely instead of abstractly. If we neglect to give our listeners a pinpointed description of behavior, they are forced to guess and infer. Specificity is an important interpersonal skill because it gives our listeners more information with which to respond. Consider the difference between these two descriptions: "He is a good employee" versus "He arrives exactly on time, never abuses his sick leave days, works overtime when needed, pursues training relevant to his job, and is consistently effective with our customers." Mutual understanding is easier when we are as specific as possible. This is a fairly straightforward example, but imagine the consequences of speaking abstractly in the heat of a conflict (Meldrum, 1986).

Abstract language makes the problem at hand seem overstated, and therefore more daunting to work to resolve. Nonspecific language gives so little information that the receiver's ability to meet the speaker's needs is greatly reduced. Abstractions beget more abstractions in return. Specific language, in contrast, prevents assumptions about what is a "given" in the discussion. We often use higher level abstractions; for instance, instead of saying: "Thanks for updating these profiles, filling those scripts, counseling the customers, and answering the phone," we would normally say: "Thanks for covering for me." Thus, we condition ourselves into speaking in a kind of shorthand that serves our purposes most of the time. But, as with ownership language, when we need to engage in a confrontation, we must be able to express ourselves in concrete behavioral terms (Deetz and Stevenson, 1986).

A behavioral description should include three components: (1) Who are the people involved? (e.g., Is your complaint directed solely at one person or does it include others?) (2) Under what circumstance does the behavior happen? (e.g., What place? What time?) (3) What behaviors are displayed? (e.g., Instead of "Stop being inconsiderate," say "I would appreciate it if you put away the spatulas and counting trays when you leave shift.") This is much better than the more common "Clean up before going home." We all know that "clean up" to one person means scrubbing, while to another it means piling, stacking, or shifting.

The skills of ownership language and specificity come together when we look at the components of responsible, assertive communication.

ASSERTIVENESS

Imagine that your boss has just asked you to stay late, without pay, to help complete a large nursing home order that should be delivered by early tomorrow morning. Coincidentally, you have tickets to the theater tonight and you have been looking forward to this production for a few weeks. What do you say?

A. "You ought to know better than to ask me to stay at the last minute. You try to use your employees to cover your mistakes."

B. "I'm so sorry, but I can't stay. My best friend is in the hospital and I promised to bring her some things she really needs. I'd be happy to stay any other night."

C. "I have important plans for the evening and I'd rather not break them. I'm sorry you're in such a bind and I'm willing to stay a few extra minutes to try to phone in some of the relief help. I hope you'll be able to finish up O.K. without me."

Each example is a refusal of the request but there are important differences among them. It is obvious which response will have the best long-term outcome.

The first response is loaded with blaming language and therefore sounds quite aggressive. This employee is quite angry and it comes out in a hostile and belittling fashion. Ironically, people who are prone to these types of outbursts have often neglected to assert themselves in the past and are now feeling too much accumulated resentment.

The second response is a good example of passive communication and may evoke sympathy and cooperation. The boss may respond, "I'm sorry to hear that, by all means go visit her," but this evades the issue at hand and weaves a lie into the working relationship. Being in the health profession, the boss is likely to ask again about the friend's "condition," the hospital she is in, and if there is anything that can be done to help. If the employee cannot cover the lie, the boss is likely to feel betrayed and no doubt will react negatively toward the employee. Not all passive messages involve a lie, but nonassertive individuals usually conceal their true feelings or predicament. Often passive communicators will capitulate and say: "Oh, I'll stay," while the manager is left in the dark about the sacrifice the employee is making. This "conditions" the boss to keep making requests, perhaps even acting on the unspoken assumption that the employee likes the overtime. Meanwhile, passive communicators build up resentments and tear down their sense of self-esteem.

The last response was an illustration of assertive communication. The employee doesn't try to justify why he is declining the request while at the same time he does show concern for the problem. If the employee offered the reason, a desperate manager might respond, "You mean a play is more important than your job?" Such a stalemate is not necessary, because the employee has the right to decline without justifying why at length.

Assertive communication is a clear and direct expression of needs, wants, and feelings. We need this skill in a wide variety of situations, such as responding negatively to requests or confronting someone about inappropriate behavior. The following guidelines should be helpful in constructing assertive messages.

In circumstances requiring assertiveness skills, it is always best not to "fly blindly" into the situation, perhaps by remembering to script yourself using the acronym C.L.E.A.R., which will prompt you to first *C*learly describe the situation as you see it. *L*isten to what the other person is saying. *E*xplain the situation specifically while expressing your feelings about it. *A*ssert your stance. *R*esults that you expect from the other person's responses are stated.

Here is what the C.L.E.A.R. system for improving assertiveness would look like if applied in a conflict situation. Example: Because of a dramatic increase in customer use of your store, there must be a redistribution of the workload. As store manager, you decide to hold a compulsory meeting to discuss with all employees how this change can be facilitated. Even though you saw Jane, a pharm tech, moments before the meeting, she did not attend. You decide to use your C.L.E.A.R. skills to talk with Jane.

- *C*lear: "A compulsory meeting was held yesterday right after we closed and although I saw you nearby a few minutes before, you did not attend."
- *L*isten: "I am ready to listen if it was because of a misunderstanding or some other reason."
- *E*xplain: "I was annoyed because without everyone there it was hard to get group consensus about the changes we need to make."
- *A*ssert: "I'd like your input and presence at the next planning meeting on Monday at 5 p.m."
- *R*esults: "If you come to the next meeting, I and the rest of the staff will appreciate it." (Positive tone for first confrontation). "If not, we will have to question your commitment to your job." (Negative tone if you have a repeated undesirable behavior pattern.)

The C.L.E.A.R. system of assertive communication incorporates the element of ownership (e.g., I was annoyed . . .) and specificity (e.g., because it is hard to get group consensus . . .) in *each* of the steps. We need to remember that the primary source of stress in our lives is our relationships. Life gets less stressful when we realize that we have the right to express our feelings and preferences in a respectful and dignified way. By carefully planning our assertive communication, we know we have done our best to package our messages in a C.L.E.A.R. and responsible manner. These skills are obviously indispensable in difficult interpersonal conflicts.

CONFLICT MANAGEMENT

What do we believe about conflict? Is it always awful or always an opportunity? Maybe we believe what Sartre once said: "Hell, it's other people," or as Thornton Wilder has claimed: "The best part of married life is the fights, the rest is merely so-so"? Often these fights that we find ourselves drawn into are symbolic of the nature of the relationship. The sum of several of these conflicts adds up to our interpersonal style and indicates whether or not we are living a burnt-out, stressed-out life.

When do our behavioral habits about conflict begin? To get a sense of how early all of this starts, we need only visit a children's playground. As we eavesdrop on the young ones at play, certain phrases are sure to sound familiar: "Quit bossing me around," "Who died and made you king?", "It's mine, I found it first," and "Mom, tell him he has to share." Twenty years later we express ourselves with "grown-up" language as we communicate in the hospital or retail store, and yet not that much has changed at all. We are still fighting over *roles* and who is pulling rank on who, and *resources*, with a constant concern about scarcity. Therefore, who will "win" becomes especially important.

Because everyone wants to be, to do, and to have, we get terribly frustrated if we feel someone is standing in our way. If people in conflict were honest about what is really going on instead of *sounding* like they are engaging in a "rational" debate, perhaps they would realize that often what is really happening is a repetitive back and forth cycle of "I could achieve my goals if you would just get out of my way," . . . "Oh yeah, well I could get what I want if you weren't holding me back." If we feel that most of the people we have conflicts with are "obstructionists," we are sure to feel defeated and exhausted most of the time.

Still, there is much about conflict that is natural, and inevitable, and can be constructive. Conflict makes us prioritize life, since most of us are not willing to fight over nothing. Conflict can sharpen decision making as it requires that we consider opposing views. Surviving conflict deepens relationships: we tend to value people that we feel free to fight with, which ultimately increases trust. A well-managed conflict resembles a productive mutual values clarification process, but a mismanaged conflict looks like a deadly duel with the goal of eliminating, neutralizing, or injuring the "opposition."

Often we get the feeling that a conflict has escalated very quickly (Meldrum, 1986). As soon as we recognize that a dispute is occurring, one and then both parties have already started to get upset. Once the people involved are upset, the disagreement becomes very personal and each side attempts to lay the blame and walk off with the last blow given. However, a battle won generally means that a war has begun, and in the retaliation phase the point of the original disagreement can be lost as each party fights to win. This phase can get pretty ugly and is reminiscent of the playground dynamics again: "Oh yeah, well what about that time in a meeting last year when you said. . . ."

What makes us escalate through these phases so quickly? Obviously, anger is the fuel that fires the liftoff and subsequently distorts our thinking processes. Anger makes us feel victimized and self-entitled, and leads us to excessive preoccupation with others' motives (e.g., "Why do they always do this to me?"). Like children who often do not seem to be able to understand the difference between negative attention and positive attention, we overstate our case and exaggerate to get attention in the heat of the moment. We become blind to how we are contributing to the problem and acquire a type of double standard thinking. Anger makes us blurt out things that are not easily forgotten or forgiven and thereby turn small differences into full blown tragedies. Anger is often masking vulnerability or what can be recognized as the "You can't fire me because I quit!" syndrome. Instead, anger should be a cue that we need to *change* not *attack* something. We need to talk to ourselves differently and say: "I can't do anything about his/her behavior. I can only behave in a better way myself."

But it is not always a matter of simply managing the anger that we manufacture inside ourselves; we also need strategies for handling the angry aggression that comes our way (sometimes quite unexpectedly). Because the person who is angry is often in a state of distorted thinking, as previously described, we need strategies to keep from getting hooked into the vicious cycle. The five basic types of responses that can be used to keep a conflict from escalating are reflective, deflective, inquiry, feedback, and deferral (Nelson-Jones, 1990).

The *reflective* response calls upon the skill of paraphrasing and restating to avoid escalation: "Sounds like you're mad because you feel that I'm not doing my share of the work," to which the other party is likely to respond: "Damn right, you aren't!" So why encourage this? This has much to do with the healing power of listening, which will be expanded on in the next section. For now, try to appreciate the fact that by not defending but also by not being aggressive ("*You feel I'm not . . .*"), you have kept the conflict from escalating. If you keep up the reflective response in combination with the other aggression management strategies, the conflict cannot escalate past the stalemate stage.

Often in conflicts the other party has a piece of the truth that needs to be acknowledged. The *deflective* response provides the option of partial agreement without self-indictment. The statement "You have a point; it can get overly busy in here" can help diffuse anger in the customer who is critical of the waiting time. Often practitioners feel as if they have to defend not only themselves but the institution for which they work. Why do we fall into this? We know and agree that our work environments are not perfect and we must remember that within reason there is some power in confirming this publicly.

At times the anger that comes our way can be overly vague: "I don't like your attitude," or "You're rude." This often shocks practitioners who are trying to do their best. Responding with an *inquiry* that invites specifics works best at these times: "What is it exactly that I did or said that upset you?" Then be prepared to listen reflectively to the emotional content of the complaint. Still, there will be times when a customer or patient is being unfairly abusive and even when you use the inquiry strategy you cannot obtain enough specific information to take corrective action. This is the time to use a *feedback* strategy: "I feel uncomfortable when you criticize me harshly without first asking my side of the story." Note the presence of ownership language and the appropriately assertive tone of the message. Trying to diffuse the anger that comes your way is not the same as being mad, gritting your teeth, and lying down while a patient or customer bulldozes over you. There is a middle ground between exploding back at them and effectively "losing it" and smiling continuously because the customer is always right.

Finally, in times of complete desperation, a *deferral* strategy may have to be used. As a consultant, the author has been told numerous stories of physical violence breaking out in the workplace, particularly between hospital co-workers. If the situation has heated up to this kind of boiling point, it is best to use a deferral strategy: "I need a little time to think about what you are saying." Contracting to talk at a later time is a last resort strategy that is infinitely better than interpersonal violence of any kind.

Whether or not we are likely to employ these aggression management strategies has a lot to do with our habitual styles in conflict situations. The four most common styles are avoidance, accommodation, competition, and compromise. A fifth under-utilized but more effective style is collaboration. A brief sketch of each follows and the cases to come will illustrate each style in greater depth (see Johnson, 1986).

People who typically avoid conflict try to deal by not dealing. They will put off having important talks, physically avoid the other party (including leaving phone calls unreturned), or psychologically withdraw even when present (that blank zombie-like look we have all witnessed). Because avoiders want immediate relief of tension they will often try to change the topic or sidestep disagreement while not appreciating the long-term buildup to which they are contributing. Avoiders don't seem to see that withholding their true opinion hurts everyone involved because they operate on a maxim of "It's not worth it." It is almost as if they believe that nothing in this world is important enough to fight for. If we are not willing to stand up for certain principles, we often experience self-esteem problems or constantly feel frustrated and devalued by others. This is clearly the case with people who are chronic conflict avoiders.

In conflicts, some people are too quick to accommodate and end up as doormats who get walked on. They try to protect the relationship by yielding, sacrificing, complying, and letting the other have his or her way. This style often seems to be a misapplication of the ethic of "turn the other cheek" as accommodators attempt to kill others with kindness, all the while thinking of themselves as the better human beings because of their efforts.

Competitors in conflict will use insults, threats, demands, and even lies if they must. Their tempers escalate quickly and sometimes they will physicalize the fight. (In fact, the author was recently told of a case where one competitive pharmacy tech broke the arm of another as he slammed him into the refrigerator in the hospital IV room.) Competitors find a way to plant the seeds of long-term ill will with very punishing strategies. They believe in standing firm and waiting for others to weaken and that people are naturally adversarial. Since they only see two kinds of people in the world, winners and losers, they naturally want to be the winner.

Compromisers represent a big improvement over the previous styles, but their shortsightedness lies in their lack of patience for the brainstorming process. They will quickly give up and try to split the difference or exchange concessions. They seem to reflect a "You scratch my back and I'll scratch yours" mentality and they figure that getting part of what they want is better than nothing. The compromiser's world view is simply not very grand, and they don't seem to appreciate the concept of "synergy" in human dialogue.

In contrast to the previous styles, collaborators are as concerned for others as they are for themselves, and tend to give and receive as much information as possible. They explore non-compromising win-win solutions in an open, creative, brainstorming fashion. Collaborators believe that truth lies in knowledge, and that we should all apply principles rather than pressure from personalities. The only thing that collaborators know for sure is that they don't know everything about the situation under discussion. They don't have preconceived ideas about what might be the best solution for a problem, and they are willing to let it emerge. Collaborators rely on reflective responses to bring down the emotional temperature of the situation so that both parties can continue to the brainstorming phase without excessive anger distorting the thinking process. Candor, honesty, and trusting behaviors typify the collaborator in action.

Even if we are using an ideal collaborative style to manage conflict, the aspects of time and place must be kept in mind. We should not start highly charged important discussions when we need to be someplace in five minutes. When dealing with a competitor, a cool-down period is sometimes necessary. An avoider will be further devastated if a confrontation of his or her behavior takes place in public where others can overhear.

In the collaborative process we must not make people stakeholders of their ideas. We can avoid win/lose dynamics by saying "The problem with that idea" versus "The problem with your idea." Patient collaboration should develop options for mutual gain, all the while keeping in mind who will ultimately benefit or lose from the resolution of the problem. As can be noted in the cases to come, when conflict is mismanaged between co-workers, it is often the patient or customer who is hurt.

In sum, in a conflict situation ask yourself, how is my anger keeping me from focusing on the principles of collaboration? Am I employing the strategies to diffuse angry aggression? What style am I using to deal or not deal with this problem? Obviously, effective listening skills are vital in resolving conflicts in a collaborative fashion.

LISTENING AND EMPATHIC COUNSELING

The sad fact is that most people do not listen most of the time. How do we know this? A few years ago, a college professor named Paul Cameron of Wayne State University conducted an experiment that required students attending a lecture to encode their thoughts and moods every time they heard a buzzer go off at sporadic intervals during class throughout the semester. Instead of listening (and there is an inherent reward for listening in this context: higher grades), about 20% of the students were pursuing erotic thoughts, another 20% were reminiscing about something, others were worrying, daydreaming, thinking about food, and so forth. On average, only 12% were actually listening to the lecture. And this was a very popular professor who was rated as a great speaker. When we think about the "inspired" little lectures that pharmacists give over and over again ("Take these three times a day with food and call your doctor if you don't feel better in three days"), we can rightly wonder how many people are actually listening. We may come to believe that the real advantage of talking to ourselves is that at least we can guarantee that someone is listening!

How did we come to be a society of such poor listeners? As was the case with behavior in conflict, poor listening starts very early in life. We all had older relatives, mothers and others that we didn't feel like listening to (still don't?), and yet our parents taught us that part of proper behavior was to sit quietly and listen whether we liked it or not. Many of us were told that we should be seen but not heard. Clearly, we didn't like it much and we would rather have been running around making noise and having fun. We were told not to be rude and to be polite and respectful. In other words, we were forced to pretend we were feeling things we really were not, and yet it was clear that to avoid our parent's anger we would minimally have to learn to "fake it." So instead of becoming good at truly listening, we have become skilled at looking and sounding as though we are listening (Anastasi, 1982). We all know how to insert a well-placed "uh-huh" into a phone conversation at just the key time that the conversational partner might suspect that we have slipped off into another activity or dimension. Many people kid themselves about their capacity to do two things at once and probably all pharmacists have attempted to read the drug index while also handling a customer's call. This is cognitively impossible! The inner voice that helps us read easily drowns out the outer voice being processed through our eardrums.

Sometimes a customer suspects that he or she has caught the pharmacist not listening because the timing on her automatic "Aha's," and "Hmmmm's," and "Yes's" is just a little bit off. The customer will test this hunch with a quick, preemptive "So what do you think?" The off-guard pharmacist can hear the trap coming deep in the recesses of her mind and is ready with "I've got to think a minute," while madly scrambling to reconstruct the conversation by recalling the bits and pieces she did hear. Because we know that we are all guilty of the same non-listening behavior at times, we will seldom try to "prove" that the other person wasn't listening through extensive entrapment. We all have been socialized into being able to look and sound as though we are listening, when in fact all we are doing is being "polite" by society's standards of acceptable behavior (Anastasi, 1982).

While this kind of faking attention and "pseudo-listening" seems to be the biggest culprit in sabotaging patient counseling, there are many other listening barriers to dismantle. In fact, the only people who might have a "good excuse" for listening difficulties are some of the very old and the very young who may have attention span deficits. The rest of us need to learn to recognize our own idiosyncratic faulty listening habits (see Adler and Rodman, 1982).

In pharmacy practice, the problem of prejudging and stereotyping the patient from physical appearance is prevalent. I know of one case where an elderly woman came in with an Rx that was written for four times daily, which she had verified verbally with her doctor when she received it. The pharmacist did not read the doctor's handwriting correctly and handed back a vial that indicated three times a day. When the elderly woman questioned the label, the pharmacist said "That's O.K. dear. I'm sure you just got a little confused," thereby failing to listen to her understanding of the instructions. Ironically, the pharmacist probably assumed that the elderly woman was not able to listen effectively to her doctor.

In workshops that the author has conducted across the country, many pharmacists have confessed that at the end of a long day, the stain on a patient's tie, a gaudy outfit, or even unusual facial hair have become a welcome, fascinating, and hypnotically transfixing distraction from whatever the patient seems to be saying. By concentrating on an irrelevant aspect of the customer's presentation of self (e.g., What a funny accent!), the pharmacist misses everything that needs to be heard.

Too often we give in to our emotional worries and preoccupations when we should be listening. Balancing a checkbook or fantasizing about going on a winning lottery megabucks spending spree in our minds diverts us away from the listening moment. Of course, the first step to better listening is closing our mouths. Woody Allen is rumored to have said "The opposite of listening is waiting"; in other words, lying in wait for the other person to take a breath, hesitate for a second, or come to the end of a sentence so that we can jump back in and dominate the conversation.

Selective listening is also a barrier because we only perk up when something of particular interest to us is mentioned. We are capable of perpetually tuning out an annoying co-worker except for those times that he may digress into "Hey, did you see the game last night?" and being big sports fans, we snap to attention. The problem with this type of listening is that when we only attend to our personal interests, we never expand the scope of our knowledge. And we are left making assumptions about the things being said because we don't truly hear all the content. Selective listening is more damaging when it is done in an "ambushing" manner. This is selective attention to the moments when the other party says something "dumb" or incorrect. In true debate style, we are case-building by stockpiling ammunition. When we think we have enough verbal munitions supplies on hand to launch an attack, we frequently start strategizing for the battle. In our heads we say "O.K., I'll start with the little grenades, move up to the bazookas, and my grand finale is dropping the big bomb.'' Meanwhile, as we plot how good we are going to sound as we use the person's own words against them, the person has been continuing to talk. We cannot hear them because the strategizing voice in our head has gotten louder than theirs. It doesn't help matters that we can think in sentences at speeds of up to 700 words per minute but can only speak at about 100 words per minute. That leaves a lot of mental room for plotting, daydreaming, and fantasizing with our inner voice.

A few additional tips for effective listening: don't tolerate distractions. Trying to place important follow-up calls when co-workers are hanging around your desk doesn't make sense. If someone uses words you don't understand, ask them for clarification rather than wondering and guessing. People want to be understood, so it is a great compliment to them to be asked for clarification. If you are too tired to listen, try to get someone to cover for you for just a few minutes so that you have a chance to regenerate a bit.

Obviously there are many benefits to be accrued from eliminating as many poor listening habits as possible. In fact, it is the author's pet theory that we can prove we are bad listeners if we need two to three people walking on the street to give us additional driving directions after we were told an extensively detailed description at the outset. This is a very simple example of lost time and effort due to poor listening habits. Imagine the consequences of taking a similar approach to listening in a phone conversation with a physician. Having to call back because we didn't get it right the first time can have a very negative personal and professional impact on us.

Becoming a better listener means being a positive influence in other people's lives. When a pharmacist continues to take shelf product inventory while at the same time talking with a customer, the customer gets the idea that "things" are a more important part of the job than connecting with people. We validate people's existence by listening to them and we thereby avoid the breakdown of the relationship. Good listeners have better vocabularies, improved performance in school or on the job, and absorb more from the world around them. Additionally, Dr. James Lynch, author of *The Language of the Heart: The Body's Response to Human Dialogue*, has conducted research that indicates that learning to be a more effective listener actually lowers blood pressure in hypertensive individuals. With all the potential benefits to be gained through better listening, it seems strange that our school systems are designed to teach writing, reading, and speaking, but not listening skills.

Once we have removed the barriers to listening, we still need to respond in such a way that the people we are with feel listened to and understood. Empathic listening is a vitally important skill because most of the counseling that goes on in our society is provided by "non-psychological" professionals. Pharmacists, doctors, nurses, lawyers, financial planners, teachers, and others end up providing most if not all of the counseling and guidance that the average American will ever receive. Professionals and paraprofessionals alike need to know a lot more than how to say "Don't worry" (Kennedy, 1977). In fact, the often used statements like "calm down" or "I know how you feel" just make the patient more upset because they feel so misunderstood by the pharmacist.

Overeducated, specialized professionals tend to see everything as a technical difficulty that can be fixed, and forget that whatever the "problem" is, there is still a sensitive human being attached. Too often pharmacists, particularly in dealing with patients on psychotropic medications, will take an automatic stance of "Hey, it isn't my business to try to relate to some of these people; it's beyond my area of expertise." This is true to a certain extent, but it is also true that even an advanced Alzheimer's patient can pick up on and internalize feelings of personal rejection because of stiff awkwardness coming from the pharmacist (Meldrum, 1990). Having empathic listening and counseling skills means that at least we do not have to increase the other person's emotional burden and that we have a very good chance of being able to lighten it. The word empathy was derived from the German word "einfuhlung" and through the Greek translation came to mean "feeling with." This is distinctly different from sympathy which means to feel sorry for an individual. Too often in the health care system patients are given doses of pseudo-sympathy that does nothing to ease their emotional distress. "Sorry, your doctor didn't call in your Rx yet," . . . "Sorry, there are no more refills on this," . . . "Sorry, but it's not my fault,"

. . . These are not psychologically satisfying responses! The health care provider sounds like an automated robot chanting these phrases hundreds of times a day.

Feeling empathy gives us an intellectual and emotional understanding of the other person's experience. It is not possible to achieve complete empathy because immersing ourselves in another person's view of the world is too difficult a task. Still, it is possible to get a sense of others' points of view and to enlist their aid in helping us refine our grasp of their reality. We don't have to agree with other people's viewpoints, we must instead understand and accept them without evaluating (Bolton, 1979).

It is easier to further define empathy by describing behaviors that are *not* empathic. Being empathic means not being judgmental, which would imply that the speaker is good or bad, right or wrong. Giving unsolicited advice, quizzing, interrogating, or placating is not responding empathically. Unfortunately, it is true that when someone "dumps" an emotional reaction on us, we are very likely to respond with one of the non-empathic responses above. Let's look at an example to see how this might play out between a speaker and listener:

> Wow, after five years of pharmacy school, I thought it was guaranteed that I could get a job right after graduation. I've been looking everywhere for a position but I can't find one. My parents always told me that after I graduated they wouldn't support me anymore. With graduation coming up next month, I'm totally overwhelmed.

Judgmental Response: "Everyone who really wants a job badly enough can get one, even if you have to work at a burger joint for a while."

Advice-Giving Response: "Network with last year's alumni, look for the posting by the pharmacy practice lab, call the general hospital's employment office."

Quizzing Response: "Have you asked the professors who teach clinical? Have you looked in the newspaper? Did you go to the career placement office?"

Placating Response: "Oh, don't worry so much, I'm sure something will turn up soon and then you'll laugh when you look back and see how silly you were to get so worked up."

Empathic Response: "Wow, with graduation right around the corner, and feeling like you can't turn to your parents one more time for help, you must be feeling incredibly stressed."

Note the mental reactions that could be likely in reaction to the five responses. The judgmental reaction would minimally provoke a "Who asked you?" or a "Get lost" type of reaction. The advice-giving response would probably provoke a "So, what, do you think I'm so stupid that I haven't already tried or thought about these things?" type of reaction. Similarly, the quizzing response communicates indirectly that even though the speaker has already said they have "looked everywhere," they somehow must have missed the basic steps of a job search that any college senior is fully capable of taking. The placating response is like getting an annoying, condescending little pat on the head. Only the empathic response speaks to the reality that is experienced by the student and is likely to provoke a further unfolding of the story: "Yeah, not only that, but my student health insurance runs out next month too!"

In reflecting the emotional state of the speaker, the listener must not only meet the other with the right kind of emotion, but also the right degree of it (Bolton, 1979). For example, if a patient says "I'm afraid this operation is just the first in an endless series of surgeries I'll have to undergo," the pharmacist may choose to respond "You sound pretty worried about this" (weak intensity), . . . "You sound quite frightened about this" (mild intensity) . . . "You sound really panicky about this" (strong intensity). At the same time they are listening for the type and intensity of emotions, pharmacists must listen with their eyes as well as their ears. The opposite of indifference is caring and a lot of concern can be communicated with a simple observation: "You look like you're not feeling too well today, is that right?"

It is important to note how easily we can compose the judgmental, advice-giving, quizzing, placating responses in our heads. Unfortunately, as we grew up, we heard an endless supply of these types of communication barriers from our family, teachers, and peers. Still, these responses serve only to block and cut off further communication, while the empathic response instead opens things up and encourages the speaker to unfold their story. Many pharmacists might counter with: "I don't have time for people to be elaborating at length with me, so I'd better not practice this empathy response." A concern for time constraints is understandable, but sometimes there is vitally important information just below the surface that must come out to avoid compliance problems or potentially tragic consequences. Also, there might be fewer follow-up and time-consuming discussions in the future because of misunderstandings that must be corrected.

It is often helpful for the pharmacist to ask a series of silent questions: "What is this person *really* saying? What can't they bring themselves to say? What are they hinting at? What are they only half saying?" For example, if a customer appears to be angry and states "I don't know why I have to pay all this money for these medications that don't work anyway," the pharmacist may respond: "Give it a chance first," or in contrast, "Sounds like you're having a hard time having faith in your treatment plan." This second statement may provoke a surprising response: "Darn right I'm skeptical! The last few drugs my doctor prescribed did me absolutely no good so I stopped taking them and felt better on my own." Obviously, by going beyond a standard advising and placating-type response, the pharmacist was given more information about the patient's likelihood of being non-compliant. Especially in the case of an increased dosage of a similar drug product, it is important to communicate with the doctor regarding the fact that the other drugs were not given a fair trial. Without empathy skills, however, none of the additional important information would have come to the surface.

Being able to practice empathy consistently and effectively has a profound effect on how we view the world. As an experiment, the author showed two of her classes the same video of two co-workers having a verbal conflict. One class was instructed to empathize with this duo as much as possible and the other class was given no instructions at all. After seeing the videotape, the class instructed to empathize was very forthcoming with possible explanations for both parties' behavior: "bad day," . . . "bad mood," . . . "stress," . . . "They don't mean to take it out on each other," . . . "It's not personal," . . . "They didn't intend to get themselves into that situation." In sharp contrast, those students who weren't reminded to be empathic said things like: "She was a real bitch," . . . "He was a bastard," . . . "People like that shouldn't work together," . . . "Maladjusted thirty-something yuppy types." In other words, those practicing empathy were more tolerant and open, and those who did not tended to make more static black and white evaluations of people's personalities.

Too frequently people learning communication skills think of empathic listening and reflective responding in conflict management (see previous section) as a type of "gimmick" to be employed in unpleasant situations. If this is the spirit behind the words, the speaker will come across as phony and untrustworthy. Becoming consistently empathic is very hard work, and it means changing your goals, not just your statements. Listening to confused, mad, sad, or scared people isn't easy. When we are with another person who is capable of being empathic we sense that it is all right to risk openness without worrying about being ridiculed, embarrassed, or shamed. Nothing horrible will happen because we revealed more about what we are thinking and feeling and there is a distinct sense that something good will come of it.

SUMMARY

We have touched upon the essential communication skills in the briefest manner possible. The driving idea behind this book is to let the case studies provide the material for learning by looking at the actual dialogue between pharmacists and their co-workers, customers, and patients.

As the case studies are analyzed, it is useful to bear in mind what we know about the barriers to effective communication, particularly those created by the pharmacist because of a level of personal defensiveness that impairs clear thinking and effective responding. Pharmacists need to ask questions in a more thoughtful and conscious way because it is all too easy to fall into a pattern of asking closed, leading questions which discourage interaction and leave the health care provider in the position of "controller."

Some situations with customers and patients require assertiveness and limit setting. At times like these, it is particularly important to use ownership language that avoids shifting the blame onto the other party. Handling and defusing angry aggression that is projected outward during conflicts is as important a skill as refraining from dispensing unfair verbal abuse. We all need to be aware of the type of interpersonal style we are likely to employ in these tough situations.

It has been established that we are a nation of poor listeners. We are skilled at looking like we are listening instead of actually listening. While appearing polite and attentive on the outside, we frequently are generating a lot of internal mental noise in our heads that drowns out the voices of the people to whom we should be listening. And even when we manage to dismantle our internal listening barriers, we often have difficulty responding in a way that helps the other person to feel understood.

For all the skills that the process of socialization heaps upon the individual, the ability to self-diagnose and self-correct communication difficulties even as they unfold is not a competence that many people manage to cultivate on their own. By analyzing the upcoming cases, pharmacists will more readily identify effective responses to challenging situations in hospital and retail practice.

PART I:
COMMUNICATION
IN THE COMMUNITY PHARMACY

At the time this text was being prepared, Ann Landers, the syndicated advice columnist, had just printed several letters about drugstore customers being shortchanged by a few pills each time they purchased a vial of medicine. Every time a story like this appears in the news, community pharmacists find themselves on the front lines with customers aggravated by whatever alarm the media has created. The task of the community pharmacist is a challenging and ongoing educational mission.

We feel we have accomplished something if we help our customers to understand that even though there is a real difference between brand name paper towels and their more coarse and unrefined generic counterparts in the supermarkets (which the customer can observe directly), there is no need to worry about such a severe quality differential with drugs. It seems that just as soon as we have our customers' trust in this respect, an investigative journalism television show will do a frightening exposé on the topic and undo the trust we have worked so hard to build.

In fact, the community pharmacist is constantly exposed to whatever "emotional baggage" customers happen to carry in with them that day. If they are worried about finances the pharmacist will probably hear about it when it comes time to pay. Many people do not even know if their health insurance covers prescriptions or not. Often patients are too intimidated to ask additional questions of their doctors and so much anxiety will accompany their statements to the pharmacist. The community pharmacist is truly the most accessible health care professional and so many "unfiltered" questions are directed to them.

Being the most public and available health care consultant is a very big job. In the era of mandatory counseling, it will be an overwhelming experience for pharmacists who cannot work well with technicians and other pharmacists. On top of this daunting task are the typical barriers in community practice that add even more pressure, e.g., time, privacy, etc. (For a complete discussion, see Tindall, Beardsley, and Kimberlin, 1989.) Challenging situations are constantly presenting themselves and quite often with very little advance warning. A retail pharmacist may have to counsel someone regarding an O.T.C. while also verifying their compliance on a long-term medication (all this, of course, while having a doctor's office on hold and a growing line of people trying to get all their errands done during lunch hour).

With such a vast array of tasks to be accomplished as part of the job, it was difficult to select case studies to illustrate what kinds of situations that the community pharmacist might face in a typical "rough" day. Therefore, no special claim is made of the "representativeness" of the scenarios that follow in Chapters 2, 3, and 4. Still, each grouping of cases should give the reader a feel for the communication options that can be chosen when in conflict with customers, counseling customers, or in confrontations with co-workers.

Chapter 2

Conflict with Customers in the Community Pharmacy

"I DON'T UNDERSTAND WHY YOU WON'T GIVE ME A REFILL"

Background

It is a busy Sunday morning on a holiday weekend at the community pharmacy. A customer arrives with a bottle with a label which states that a new prescription is needed for a refill. Robin has to handle an irritated Mr. Faber who suffers occasional attacks of gout.

[Robin's unspoken thoughts are italicized and set off by brackets.]

Mr. Faber: "I'd like to have this prescription refilled."

Robin: [*Here we go.*] "I'll be happy to check that for you . . . (notices no refill label) I'm sorry, sir, this cannot be refilled."

Mr. Faber: "Yes it can. I've had it filled before." *— must assume hers ignorant*

attribution theory

Robin: [*He isn't going to listen. Keep cool.*] "I'll check our files. It says here that your physician only wrote for one refill and you've had it already."

Mr. Faber: "That doesn't mean anything; the boss has been filling it for me."

attributing

Robin: [*That's a lie. The file says this has been refilled only once.*] "Your prescription has only been refilled once. I'll give you enough to get through Tuesday, but then you have to call your doctor."

ordering

33

Mr. Faber: "I don't understand why you won't give me a refill."

Robin: [*Is this guy dumb?*] "This label indicates that your physician requested only one refill."

Mr. Faber: "Like I said, the label doesn't mean anything."

Robin: [*Is he crazy?*] "The label means a lot; it is the result of federal legislation."

Mr. Faber: "What's the difference? The boss fills it all the time."

Robin: [*He wants me to break the law and he's lying.*] "Look, legally I can't fill it. I don't plan on losing my license because you don't believe in following the law." [*I didn't want to lose my temper.*]

Mr. Faber: "Just give me enough 'til Tuesday. I still don't understand what the big deal is."

Robin: [*He is dense. I'm going to make him understand why I'm not refilling his prescription.*] "Why don't you understand? The law is the law. Besides, your doctor wrote one refill for a reason."

Mr. Faber: "Just give me that bottle. See you later."

Case Commentary

What Happened?

Although Robin is probably a very dedicated professional, she came across as cold and uncaring. Robin acts in a burnt-out and angry manner in this situation, and perhaps it is because she doesn't feel listened to. Often we feel like people aren't listening to us when they simply are not agreeing with us. The pharmacist missed a good opportunity to explain the value of reassessing drug therapy before committing to the long-term administration of one treatment. Robin probably wanted the customer to appreciate that the label was there to protect therapeutic outcomes. What kept these people from responding effectively to each other?

How Did Unspoken Thoughts and Assumptions Affect the Interaction?

Robin attributed many negative motivations to the customer. The progression of blaming in her unspoken dialogue is really quite striking. The customer goes from being a bad listener, to being stupid, then crazy, and finally to being a criminal. Robin does not allow for mistakes and slowness in understanding, and by the end of their "consultation," Robin just wants to know how she can *make* (force) him to understand. The spirit of "helping" him was long lost. Robin also seems to assume throughout the conversation that she is expressing her reasoning clearly enough to be instantly understood; yet she never does follow through with a complete explanation of why the policy exists. She assumes the man is trying to bully and intimidate her, rather than responding in desperation to a flare-up of his gout.

How Did the Communication Strategies Affect the Outcome?

By going immediately to the issue of law and license as the reason for saying no, the pharmacist missed a good opportunity to provide health care education. At no point did the pharmacist break away from her repetitive statements to ask if Mr. Faber was in pain. Robin never asked any questions about how Mr. Faber thought his drug therapy was going. Although all professionals realize that good customer service means keeping tempers in check, Robin did become rather sarcastic. Because this situation degenerated into a control struggle, Mr. Faber will not feel as if he is taking an active part in his treatment. Robin came across like an automaton, rigidly repeating the same defense over and over again. She is in control by virtue of the fact that she can dispense or not dispense. Why continue to act as if Mr. Faber is an enemy that must be beaten down?

How Could This Have Been Handled Differently?

What keeps people from breaking away from a vicious cycle of negative debate once they are in the thick of it? What kept Robin from saying: "I sound like a broken record; can we start over because it seems as if we are having a hard time understanding each other?" The attention needs to be focused on the communication breakdown rather than who will "win out." Robin also made a big mistake by failing to address Mr. Faber's feelings first and foremost. She needed to validate his reality by saying something like:

"I can see that you're frustrated by not being able to get your prescription when you thought there would be no problem." Also, taking additional ownership in this case might help: "I'm sorry if it wasn't made clear to you when you were in last time that this was your last refill." Note that this is not an indictment of the counseling skills of everyone on staff; it is simply an acknowledgment that misunderstandings can and do happen.

Robin needed to share more of her professional knowledge in an accessible style. She should have said: "In the past, when this doctor has written for only one refill, it was because he wanted to talk again with his patient to make sure the drug and dosage were working." This type of statement also needed to be made toward the beginning of the conversation and not later on at the point when people are unwilling to listen. Robin and all retail pharmacists on the "front lines" every day need to learn to be more empathic and less defensive.

(For more details on this case study, see Meldrum and Rando, 1987.)

"I CAN'T WAIT. I'M GOING TO BE LATE FOR CHURCH"

Background

It's late Saturday afternoon around four. Lots of customers are lined up at Neighborhood Drug, Inc. An older man makes his way through the line and demands attention. He complains about the service in a loud voice.

[John's unspoken thoughts are italicized and set off by brackets.]

Mr. St. Clair: "I've been waiting so long; can't anyone wait on me?"

John: "Thank you. (taking vials) That will be 15 minutes."

Mr. St. Clair: "What do you mean? Mass starts at 4:30. I can't wait that long!"

John: [*I'm sick of these cranks!*] "Sorry. Other people were here first. I'll do my best."

Mr. St. Clair: "I never have to wait when George is working."

John: "Sorry, but this is a busy time. How about coming by to get them after church?"

Mr. St. Clair: "No, I can wait five minutes now."

John: "I said that 15 minutes was the best I could do." [*He knows what I said.*]

Mr. St. Clair: (four minutes later) "Are my pills ready yet? I can't wait; I'm going to be late for church. How long could it take to count pills? Where is George–he doesn't make me wait."

John: [*I can't wait to get rid of you! Pain in the rear!*] "I'm starting on yours now. It will just be a little while."

Mr. St. Clair: "Christ! You mean you haven't even started yet? What have you been doing?"

John: [*What do you think I've been doing?*] "I told you before, filling the prescriptions of people in front of you. You have to be patient."

Mr. St. Clair: "Give me my bottles back, I'm coming back when George is on. My God, I can't wait forever for you."

John: (handing back bottles) "Yes, you'd better deal with George from now on." [*Leave before I swear at you.*]

Case Commentary

What Happened?

This is an all too familiar scenario for the pharmacist. If the "saintly" customer isn't on his way to church, he is usually about to catch a plane, or has a cab out front with the meter on. Rush, rush, rush! What's so complicated? Throw those pills in this bottle! Right? Wrong!

Pharmacists in this situation are frequently torn between trying to "teach the customer a lesson"–that he or she isn't the only person on earth with needs–or genuinely trying to work as quickly as possible in order to be helpful (or get rid of the individual). Many customers will directly or indirectly try to rush the pharmacist without thinking about the possible consequences of such pressure (e.g., mistakes, lack of receptivity to medication questions). It is up to the pharmacist to interrupt this process so that the exchange will remain pleasant and productive.

How Did Unspoken Thoughts and Assumptions Affect the Interaction?

John certainly doesn't have even one charitable thought about our good churchgoer. How might the interaction have gone differently if he had stopped to look at the situation in a different way? What if he had said to himself: "Older folks sometimes have a harder time getting around; I'll bet it would be hard for him to make a second trip back," or simply, "I wonder why he seems so desperate?" Did John assume that the patient needed each of his refills completed right at that moment? Would Mr. St. Clair have been pleased if John had offered enough meds to hold him over the weekend so he could come back when it was convenient? Was there any other way to handle this? Of course, creative problem solving doesn't have a chance when all of our energy is drained off by silent name-calling.

How Did the Communication Strategies Affect the Outcome?

What if all of Mr. St. Clair's huffing and puffing really meant that he was mad at himself for not allowing enough time to get his drugs and get to church also? By the time John got around to offering the constructive suggestion of having him come back after church, it was really too late to compromise; the negativity was already too strong.

From Mr. St. Clair's point of view, John never expressed even one word of understanding. John repeatedly said that he was "sorry," but we all have been in customer service situations where we know that the worker is saying "sorry" in a totally unbelievable, perfunctory, unfeeling manner. We hardly hear the sympathy in a genuine "sorry" that *is* genuine, since it is usually empathy we crave anyway.

How Could This Have Been Handled Differently?

In addition to acknowledging that Mr. St. Clair was in a rush, John could also have inquired as to whether all the prescriptions needed to be filled immediately. It could have been possible that Mr. St. Clair only needed one prescription right away, and he could have come back at a more convenient time for the others. It would be helpful if John resisted getting "reactive" to the customer's comments regarding the other pharmacist. Perhaps if John had given Mr. St. Clair a little more empathy, Mr. St. Clair would not have minded waiting, or he might not have been as impatient. Customers are not interested in hearing other people's problems; they are only interested in their own. John should not have tried the "It's very busy here and there are customers waiting in line in front of you . . ." statement. Mr. St. Clair probably interpreted it as John saying that his order wasn't important. Still, having other customers to serve is stressful. Mr. St. Clair needs to be made aware of the problem. John could say: "I'm in a bit of a bind here, Mr. St. Clair. While I can see that you're desperate to get your prescription filled, I feel obligated to first help the customer who came in before you. I'll work as quickly as possible." It is important that John responds to Mr. St. Clair by presenting a realistic picture while at the same time not dismissing his needs.

"ARE CYTOMEL AND CYTOXAN THE SAME THING?"

Background

Tim is covering the bench at a small independent pharmacy. A women calls to say that she picked up a prescription that was supposed to be for Cytoxan and upon getting home noticed that the vial was labeled Cytomel. She wants to know if this is a mistake, and if so, who filled the Rx.

[Tim's unspoken thoughts are italicized and set off by brackets.]

Mrs. Walsh: "I had my prescription filled there today. Are Cytomel and Cytoxan the same thing?"

Tim: "No. Why are you asking? Is there a problem?"

Mrs. Walsh: "My prescription was filled there and the doctor said I was to get Cytoxan but my bottle label says Cytomel. I must have the wrong thing!"

Tim: [*Oh no, major problem.*] "Can I have your name and address to double-check your profile and prescription? Hang on a minute. . . I checked it against your original prescription. If you can come in we can take care of it for you."

Mrs. Walsh: "You mean that I have the wrong drug? What if I hadn't noticed; these could have killed me!"

Tim: [*This is a huge, stupid mistake! I'm glad I didn't do it.*] "Mrs. Walsh, I can assure you nothing bad would have happened. Come in and we'll take care of it."

Mrs. Walsh: "I want to know who did this! I made an extra trip to town and now I have to come again? I'm going to speak with Henry (owner and pharmacist) about who is responsible."

Tim: [*I'd be mad but she's really over the edge. Oh no, these are Henry's initials. She's really raving mad.*] "I don't think you need to know who did it. I'll make sure the whole staff knows about the mistake."

Mrs. Walsh: "Who filled my pills?"

Tim: [*You asked for this.*] "Okay, Henry did. Do you want me to call him at home to tell him about it?" [*I'm going to have to let Henry know.*]

Mrs. Walsh: "I'm coming right in to straighten this out. I know that Henry wouldn't have made this mistake."

Tim: "I'm afraid Henry did fill it; you will have to direct your complaint to him."

(Tim calls Henry.)

Tim: [*You messed up.*] "Henry, you made a prescription mistake with Mrs. Walsh and she is very upset. She's on her way back to the pharmacy."

Henry: "I remember it exactly; I couldn't have done it wrong!"

Tim: [*Admit it already. How are you going to get out of this? She's furious!*] "She read the label and it didn't match the original Rx. You should probably be here when she comes in."

Henry: "I'm on my way."

Case Commentary

What Happened?

If Tim's objective was to keep the customer from panicking and to maintain her faith in the pharmacy, he didn't manage to achieve either. Obviously, if the customer is on Cytoxan she is having serious health problems and is probably already feeling burdened by her health care needs. Tim mishandled not one, but two people in this case. Not only did he fail to empathize with Mrs. Walsh, but Henry also probably lost a lot of confidence in Tim's ability to handle things alone. Tim will have to work hard to restore his credibility with both people.

How Did Unspoken Thoughts and Assumptions Affect the Interaction?

Tim assumed the patient would be upset if she realized the magnitude of the mix-up and he sought to keep from revealing that information to her. Most people can sense when they are being "managed" or lied to by omission and it makes them feel manipulated.

Tim has a number of thoughts racing through his mind. He is grateful that he didn't make the mistake. He knows he would be angry too and yet he quickly tires of Mrs. Walsh's anger. Why is it that we have infinitely more patience for our own emotional states than the feelings of others? Tim's assumption that he had to protect Henry prolonged an inevitable confrontation and created more bad feelings. Tim's attitude toward Henry communicated that mistakes are something that no one likes to admit and that thinking undoubtedly affected how he broke the news to Henry. Why did Tim instantly assume that the best way to support his boss and be a team player was to try to pacify the customer without telling her the whole truth?

How Did the Communication Strategies
Affect the Outcome?

Tim decided to use an indirect communication strategy with Mrs. Walsh. She asked him if she had the wrong drug and he never said "Yes," just, "Come in and we'll take care of it for you." He tells her that nothing would have happened to her but he *never* acknowledges the reality that, although the wrong drug may not have hurt her badly, she still would be taking a substance that would not be therapeutic for her actual disease state. He was indirectly acknowledging: "It's not fatal, but it's sure not going to help you feel better." If the mistake wasn't discovered in a timely fashion, her condition would have worsened. Tim was willing to be the one to fix the problem, but apparently he didn't even want to offer apologies and possible reparations on behalf of the pharmacy.

Tim also mishandled Henry. He opened the conversation by telling Henry he had made a mistake. This made it seem like he was dumping and blaming with a "better you than me buddy" attitude. He should have opened with a collaborative "we have a problem" approach. By not leading with such strong blaming language, Henry may have felt free to admit his mistake. Every pharmacist knows that Rx mistakes are incredibly dreaded and guilt-inducing. Why make it worse?

How Could This Have Been Handled Differently?

Tim needed to start by acknowledging Mrs. Walsh's horror. He could have said something like: "I guess this has given you quite a scare, hasn't it? I'm so glad you were cautious enough to notice the difference." If the patient persists in expressing her anger, the pharmacist needs to be willing to go through the cycle. By continuing to say things like "I can hear that you're upset," and staying with these empathic, reflective strategies, the conflict does not get the fuel to escalate. As soon as Mrs. Walsh realizes she is being listened to, she'll calm down and she may no longer have the urge to storm the store. A free delivery of the correct medication could be offered as partial compensation. Mrs. Walsh felt doubly wronged by having to make two trips and there is no need to put this extra salt in the wound.

Tim seemed to take personal offense from the fact that Mrs. Walsh couldn't believe that Henry filled her prescription. It is almost as if every time that she said "Henry wouldn't do it," Tim heard her accusing him personally. Why internalize this? Why not agree with her at least in part, by saying "It is shocking that Henry would make a mistake; he is an excellent pharmacist and a very responsible person. I know he is going to feel very bad about this." By saying something along these lines, Tim reduces the chances that Mrs. Walsh will come flying into the store with retaliation on her mind. Ironically, simply telling more of the truth, and trying not to hide information would have helped the situation immeasurably.

"I WANT THE BRAND NAME AND THAT'S FINAL!"

Background

It is Thursday afternoon at a local independent pharmacy during a busy Christmas week. Lots of folks are buying cold and flu remedies. A customer approaches and hands over a prescription.

[Dan's unspoken thoughts are italicized and set off by brackets.]

Mr. Poole: "Hi, can you fill this Valium prescription for me?"

Dan: [*Great, more work.*] "Sure, that will be about fifteen minutes."

Mr. Poole: "That's okay."

(later)

Dan: "Here you go." [*He seems okay.*]

Mr. Poole: "Thank you and Merry Christmas."

(an hour later)

Dan: "Mr. Poole, what are you doing back again?"

Mr. Poole: "You gave me Diazepan when my script said Valium; are you stupid?"

Dan: [*He's angry that I gave him the generic.*] "Let me double-check."

Mr. Poole: "Yeah, you'd better."

Dan: "It seems that your physician wrote for the generic; he did not specify brand name."

Mr. Poole: "I saw the paper with my own eyes."

Dan: [*I'll try to reason but he won't understand.*] "Do you know that the generic is saving you $9.50?"

Mr. Poole: "I don't care about the measly $9.50; the doctor wrote Valium for a reason."

Dan: [*He has no clue about generics.*] "Generics are the same as the brand name."

Mr. Poole: "I know what generics are, I'm not stupid. I want the brand name and that's final. So give me the drug or just give me back the prescription paper."

Dan: [*I'm angry.*] "If you go to any other pharmacy they will tell you the same thing. So stop being irrational so we can get you on your way."

Mr. Poole: "I don't understand why you're being this way but I guess I have to take what you have."

Dan: [*Phew!*] "There you go."

Mr. Poole: "Bye."

Dan: "Can you let me explain why I had to act like this and that it isn't personal." /

Mr. Poole: "Forget it."

Case Commentary

What Happened?

Dan had the objective of helping the patient to understand what it means when a prescription is *not* marked "no substitution." Either Dan or the customer would have to contact the doctor to dispense the brand name. Mr. Poole was very unhappy about receiving the generic of Valium and Dan tried to argue as to why he should be satisfied. Mr. Poole left on a very sour note without having learned enough about generics or the state law that dictated Dan's action.

How Did Unspoken Thoughts and Assumptions Affect the Interaction?

Dan believed throughout the encounter that the patient "won't understand" and that he has "no clue." This belief lead Dan to give the information about generics in a condescending way and Mr. Poole clearly resented the implication that he didn't know what a generic was. Dan decided that Mr. Poole was being unreasonable and therefore let himself "off the hook" in terms of accepting the burden of trying to communicate with Mr. Poole. Dan continued to assume that Mr. Poole simply didn't or couldn't understand when in fact he was saying that he understood but wanted it to not be true or changed immediately. Dan further assumed that by holding out the carrot of money saved, all of Mr. Poole's concerns would simply disappear.

How Did the Communication Strategies Affect the Outcome?

Dan had some very basic listening problems in this case. Mr. Poole said: "I saw the paper with my own eyes" (meaning, "I believed I would get what it said–Valium"). Dan said: "You save $9.50," which does not address the customer's issue about not getting what he expected. Why not validate that he must have been a bit shocked and taken aback? Mr. Poole said he didn't care about the money and Dan proceeded to tell him *why* he was saving money that he didn't care about.

By the time Dan laid it on the line and told him that he was stuck ("Any other pharmacy will tell you the same"), it came out in a "Tough luck, you lose" punitive fashion. In the end, Dan seemed to start to feel guilty but then didn't know how to begin to mend the gap that had been created.

How Could This Have Been Handled Differently?

Dan needed to step out of the competitive style that he fell into with this patient. When Mr. Poole come storming in insulting Dan's intelligence, he could have said: "I feel uncomfortable being criticized so harshly without first being allowed to explain my actions." He could have validated the customer's concerns: "I can see that you've got your mind made up about getting the brand name and many other folks feel exactly like you do, except it presents a bit of a problem for *us* in this case." Dan could then present a uniform prescription blank and say "Although it's hard to notice this when reading the prescription tablet, the "no substitution" box is left unchecked . . . . The only way we can change this is if you decide to call your doctor for a new Rx." Most importantly, Dan needed to tell Mr. Poole that it was reasonable to assume what he did and that it is shocking not to get what he expected. Many customers need extra education about generics because when they buy generic paper towels in the supermarket they can see with their eyes that the quality is often not as good as the brand name. Because they are not able to examine the pharmaceutical production process, customers may have lingering doubts about the difference that need to be addressed.

"BUT I SAW ON TV HOW YOU CAN TRANSFER PRESCRIPTIONS BY SATELLITE AND COMPUTER!"

Background

It was Monday evening at Valued Consumer Store and after stocking six cartons of drugs and filling over 150 prescriptions, Beth couldn't wait until closing time in 20 minutes. A customer comes in for a birth control refill.

[Beth's unspoken thoughts are italicized and set off by brackets.]

Ms. Brown: "Can I have this refilled?"

Beth: [*Great timing, I love working past shift's end.*] "Sure, that should be ten minutes . . . (As customer hands over compact, Beth notices that it is for another store.) I'm sorry, but I can't refill this."

Ms. Brown: "But you just told me you could."

Beth: [*She's gonna be angry, let me explain.*] "You got this from another store and I need your doctor's permission to transfer it here."

Ms. Brown: "But I saw it on TV, how I could walk into any of the stores in this chain and you'd transfer the prescription by satellite and computer!"

Beth: [*Too much TV on her brain.*] "The small disclaimer at the end of the ad says that this state is not allowed to do the transfers like that."

Ms. Brown: "I can't understand why you just can't fill this now."

Beth: [*She's stubborn.*] "The law does not permit me to."

Ms. Brown: "So what am I supposed to do?"

Beth: "I can contact your doctor tomorrow for you."

Ms. Brown: "Just give me my compact back."

Beth: [*I'm too tired to be sweet.*] "Are you sure?"

Ms. Brown: "Yeah, I'll go to a real store tomorrow."

Case Commentary

What Happened?

Beth wanted to be helpful to the customer but her hands were tied. She also wanted to persuade Ms. Brown to allow her to call the doctor as a customer service but by the time she offered to do so, the situation was hard to turn around. Both customer and pharmacist were feeling the pressure since it was ten minutes to closing.

How Did Unspoken Thoughts and Assumptions Affect the Interaction?

Upon first seeing that the patient had a common birth control compact, Beth led her to believe that there would be no problem (even at that late hour) in getting a refill. All pharmacists need to be careful about situations like this when accepting refill containers from walk-ins. It only takes a second or two to build expectations and hopes. Nobody likes to feel "jerked around" and customers may actually believe that pharmacists act on whims rather than policy. Maybe Ms. Brown thought that Beth didn't want to risk working past quitting time. Even if these attributions of negative motivation only stay in customer's minds for a moment, it is enough to affect the tone and choice of words being uttered.

But it was not just the expectations set up by her first contact with Beth that shaped Ms. Brown's behavior. She arrived with the idea that in the satellite age, any branch of Valued Consumer Store in the country (and maybe Canada) could meet her needs as efficiently as any other. The fact is that pharmacy practice is not yet and never will be as "user-friendly" as the ubiquitous automated teller machines, and yet a series of nationalized pharmacy TV ads give the less critical consumer that exact impression. (Pity the pharmacist working in the branch store by the airport. Customers think they can pop by for a refill or two right before boarding that international flight.)

Ms. Brown is not being unreasonable in assuming that a woman over 18 should have no problems obtaining birth control pills. What she does not think about (and Beth is no help in this regard) is that many drugs cannot and should not be allowed universal transferability. For example, what would happen to the maintenance of records on restricted schedule drugs if the location of a patient's profile kept moving? Beth misses out on her opportunity to enlighten Ms. Brown and correct her misinformed assumptions.

How Did the Communication Strategies Affect the Outcome?

Beth used a communication strategy *very common* among pharmacists. She relied on reciting "the law" as the reason why she could not give the refill and she never did state why the law is needed in the first place. This preoccupation with law and policy often keeps pharmacists from seeming human and compassionate. Rarely do we see a case in which the pharmacist at least says: "You know, I wish I could refill this for you. . . ."

Although Beth keeps herself from being directly discourteous, she is not exactly sympathetic either. With communication in these types of settings, it is difficult to figure out which person is the most incompetent communicator. Did Beth's lack of empathy cause Ms. Brown's pushy statements or did Ms. Brown's snippiness put Beth off?

How Could This Have Been Handled Differently?

Did Beth have the option of giving Ms. Brown enough birth control medication for that evening? Would that have made this customer more willing to have her doctor called in the morning? How about some basic empathy: "I know it's a pain to have rushed down here before closing only to find it was a wasted trip. I'm sorry that the TV ads were not more clear. . . . I know that when a woman is on regular birth control the last thing she wants to hear is that it can't be refilled."

Ironically, during the time spent in the pointless back and forth conversation, Beth could have called the other V.C.S. across town and Ms. Brown might have gotten her refill before closing. Instead, Beth goes home feeling bad and the store has lost another customer.

Chapter 3

Counseling Customers in the Community Pharmacy

"THANKS FOR TALKING WITH ME"

Background

It is noontime at an urban store and Terry tries to be helpful to a local police officer trying to buy some O.T.C.s.

[Terry's unspoken thoughts are italicized and set off by brackets.]

Terry: "Can I help you?" [*He looks under the weather.*]

Mr. Kreckler: "I'm not feeling well."

Terry: "What seems to be the problem?"

Mr. Kreckler: "I have a cough and a runny nose; it feels like a cold."

Terry: [*Could be a number of things.*] "What other symptoms do you have?"

Mr. Kreckler: "Itchy eyes."

Terry: "How long have you been feeling this way?"

Mr. Kreckler: "About three days."

Terry: "Did you have the itchy eyes before the other symptoms?"

Mr. Kreckler: "Come to think of it, yes."

Terry: [*I've got a hunch about this.*] "Tell me about your work environment."

Mr. Kreckler: "I'm a cop and I've been doing extra duty down by the Charlestown waterfront construction site. With all the blasting, I'm surprised I haven't gone deaf."

Terry: [*Lots of allergens in the air.*] "What happens when they blast?"

Mr. Kreckler: "I keep people back while they make holes for the foundation. Traffic can't move until the smoke clears."

Terry: "Have you or anyone in your family had allergies?"

Mr. Kreckler: "My kids get shots for allergies."

Terry: [*Bingo!*] "It seems like you might not have a cold but that you are having an allergic reaction to the dust smoke–when that smoke gets in your eyes, your body's reaction is to try to flush it out by producing liquids, which is probably why you have the runny nose and phlegm. Are you taking any other kinds of medication right now?"

Mr. Kreckler: "No."

Terry: [*Hope this helps.*] "I think an antihistamine should take care of your temporary symptoms. If not, see your doctor."

Mr. Kreckler: "Thanks for talking with me; I would have bought the wrong stuff."

Case Commentary

What Happened?

In countries other than the United States, the neighborhood pharmacist frequently acts more like a nurse practitioner who is empowered to do elementary diagnosis and prescribe from certain classes of drugs as well as recommend O.T.C.s. In the case of Terry and Mr. Kreckler, we encounter a similar situation where the pharmacist acts as a more holistic practitioner. Good communication skills are needed to determine if the customer's problems can be helped by O.T.C.s or if they require a physician's expertise.

How Did Unspoken Thoughts and Assumptions Affect the Interaction?

The progression of Terry's unspoken thoughts makes it seem like she is a detective following up on some hot leads. It is almost as if we can see Terry working through a mental decision tree to arrive at the most likely conclusion. Still, by deliberately staying open at the beginning of the discussion, she reminds herself that different medical conditions sometimes have similar symptom patterns. Terry's genuine desire to involve herself in trying to be helpful is evident from the progression of her thoughts. It is true, as Mr. Kreckler said, that he would have bought the wrong O.T.C. had it not been for Terry's thoughtfulness. It may seem easier in the moment to let the customer buy any product he or she seems inclined to buy (usually the cheapest), but that does not mean they will be satisfied and perceive the pharmacist as a competent, caring professional.

How Did the Communication Strategies Affect the Outcome?

The careful reader of this text may get the idea that reflective empathic listening is always a good first response to any customer, patient, or co-worker who expresses some type of physical or mental discomfort. Reflective empathic listening is *usually* a good first response, but certainly not always. In this case, if Terry had given an initial response of "Sounds like you think you've got quite a bad cold," it would have served to lead both pharmacist and patient down the wrong avenue. Mr. Kreckler would have probably said something like: "I think so" to the reflective response and not elaborated further. Unfortunately, at this point it would be easy for the pharmacist to fall into asking a few more closed-ended questions and then bag the wrong O.T.C. for the sale.

diagnose and prescribe

How Could This Have Been Handled Differently?

Terry did a good job with Mr. Kreckler, so there is not a lot of advice to give. If the pharmacist had lapsed into the usual series of closed-ended questions, the customer would have felt defensive and unequal in the conversation. By responding in kind only to closed questions, Mr. Kreckler would have felt compelled to speak only when spoken to, would have worried about speaking out of turn and would have believed that the pharmacist knows best and has already decided what to do and is merely confirming the diagnosis. Instead, Terry asked five open-ended questions (note the inquiries beginning with "what," "how," and "tell me about") and then followed up with three necessary and specific probing closed-ended questions (note the inquiries beginning with "did," "have," and "are"). Since the open-ended questions yielded good information, the closed questions allowed the pharmacist to use her knowledge to identify the problem and suggest a solution. Terry also gives Mr. Kreckler a clear and detailed explanation for why he could logically conclude that he had the symptoms of a cold. Both pharmacist and customer can go away feeling good about the quality of service provided.

"CAN'T YOU SEE I HAVE A SICK CHILD?"

Background

Kirk is on duty in a small local pharmacy. A woman had brought in a prescription that was to be filled while she was out doing errands. There is a problem because the medication was discontinued. The customer returns to pick up the medication for her sick child.

[Kirk's unspoken thoughts are italicized and set off by brackets.]

Kirk: "May I help you?"

Mrs. Jay: "I'm here to get Billy Jay's medicine."

Kirk: [*She's going to be upset.*] "When I tried to fill your prescription, I noticed that it was written for a medication that is no longer made by the manufacturer."

Mrs. Jay: "What do you mean? Can't you see I have a sick child? What am I supposed to do?"

Kirk: [*I can only try my best.*] "When I noticed the problem I asked myself what I could do to help."

Mrs. Jay: "You'd better. It's your job and my baby is sick."

Kirk: [*Resist taking the bait.*] "I consulted my drug index and found a medication that is identical to the one your doctor prescribed. We have it in stock."

Mrs. Jay: "Are you sure?"

Kirk: [*This seems to be working.*] "100% positive; and I've recalculated the dosage because it is a different medication with a different concentration per dosage and because your baby is so small."

Mrs. Jay: "Did you ok this with my physician?"

Kirk: [*She doesn't trust me.*] "I'm in the process of doing that as we speak. I have a call in to her and I'm waiting for a call back."

Mrs. Jay: "Well, ok then."

Kirk: [*We're in the clear.*] "Why don't you leave me your phone number and I'll call you as soon as everything is set. That way you won't have to wait around."

Mrs. Jay: "That would be great and you don't have to rush the job because the doctor gave me some medication to use for a few days."

Kirk: "No problem, glad I could help."

Mrs. Jay: "Thank you for your efforts."

Kirk: [*Crisis averted.*] "You're welcome. Have a good evening."

Case Commentary

What Happened?

This is an excellent example of collaborative problem-solving skills in action. Kirk took positive, proactive steps to minimize the problem and hoped that Mrs. Jay would recognize the effort being put forth. Unfortunately, the customer didn't come to appreciate Kirk until the end of the conversation and in fact she actively "baited" him a few times during their interaction. Kirk managed to remain effective and avoided lapsing into negative, reactive behavior. Although he could have improved his behavior with a little more noticeable empathy, he did well to keep a potentially explosive situation from escalating.

*How Did Unspoken Thoughts and Assumptions
Affect the Interaction?*

Kirk assumes from the beginning that Mrs. Jay is going to be upset and thereby resolves to come right out with the bad news instead of trying to ease in with it and paradoxically make things worse. The pharmacist is employing a two-part strategy of making an extra effort to solve the problem while resisting automatic responses to Mrs. Jay's emotionally charged remarks. Instead of being insulted by Mrs. Jay's lack of trust, Kirk chooses to find it to be an understandable reaction and plans accordingly to get additional reassurance from her doctor to pass along. Notice Kirk's relief when he realizes that his communication skills have really worked to help the situation.

How Did the Communication Strategies Affect the Outcome?

Of course the situation would have been managed more smoothly if Mrs. Jay had been called earlier and had not made a wasted trip with her sick baby in tow. Kirk states explicitly, "When I noticed the problem I asked myself what I could do to help." Although Mrs. Jay is not quite yet in the mood to appreciate his efforts, this statement does at least keep the dialogue open. Kirk then uses positive, action-oriented language to describe all he has done and will do for Mrs. Jay. Upset customers simply want the problem fixed so that they won't get hurt in the process. Kirk's detailed explanation of the steps he has taken gives Mrs. Jay that reassurance. Because Mrs. Jay comes to believe in Kirk's sincerity, she freely offers the information about having some samples to tide her over until Kirk can get the O.K. If people are mad and typically see the other person as the enemy or someone to be punished, they will withhold helpful information (like the fact that she had the samples from the doctor) to further pressure and "guilt-trip" the person with whom they are in conflict.

How Could This Have Been Handled Differently?

Kirk handled Mrs. Jay fairly well but could do a few more things to improve the next time a similar situation occurs. Mrs. Jay's remark early on in the conversation, "Can't you see I have a sick child?" indicates she doesn't feel an adequate amount of verbal or nonverbal empathy coming from the pharmacist. Initially Kirk leaves Mrs. Jay hanging a bit when he makes his comment about the drug no longer being made. Perhaps he should have added "And that worried me because I know your child isn't feeling well and I want him to get the medicine he needs as soon as possible." Instead of waiting for Mrs. Jay to ask, Kirk could have anticipated: "I thought you might be concerned about switching your child's medication, so I want you to know that after I found a substitute and recalculated the dosage I put in a call to your doctor to check this all out." Because Kirk was able to show his efforts and competence, Mrs. Jay was able to settle down enough to listen and realize she was getting the help she needed.

"WHAT MEDICATION AM I TAKING?"

Background

A seventy-five-year-old woman with some type of organic dementia enters the pharmacy. Louise must try to verify that she understands how to take her medicine.

[Louise's unspoken thoughts are italicized and set off by brackets.]

Louise: "May I help you?" [*She looks a little shaky.*]

Mrs. O'Clair: "Oh, am I in the pharmacy?" (She is holding Rx bottle.)

Louise: "You are in the pharmacy."

Mrs. O'Clair: "Oh, I guess I am. I get lost sometimes when I go walking with my dog."

Louise: [*No dog in sight.*] "That sounds a little scary. I'll be happy to fill your prescription if you'll give me the bottle in your hand."

Mrs. O'Clair: "What medication am I taking?"

Louise: [*I know how to deal with these people.*] "Mrs. O'Clair, you are taking _____ . I'm going to fill this bottle and give it back to you."

Mrs. O'Clair: "Ok."

Louise: "I'm going to write out the name of your drug, the number, and how many times a day you will be taking it."

Mrs. O'Clair: "What are you talking about?"

Louise: [*I'd better look for reinforcements.*] "It seems to me that you are frightened and alone. I'd like to give you a special pill box with a timer, but I'd also like to explain about your medication to one of your friends or relatives. Can you give me the name of someone you live with?"

Mrs. O'Clair: "I live with my daughter."

Louise: [*I'd better follow up on this.*] "Okay, I'm going to call her so she also understands about your medication. I'm also writing out my name and phone number. Call me if you're not sure how to take your medication."

Case Commentary

What Happened?

   It appears that Mrs. O'Clair is suffering from some kind of organic dementia. To verify that this is the case, Louise needs to do more than guess by inferring from her prescription medication. Louise needs to do a more formal assessment of Mrs. O'Clair's functioning so that she can channel this information to her family, doctor, or other caregivers. Although the pharmacist did pretty well at managing the customer's anxious emotional state, more could have been done to respond specifically to her dementia-induced cognitive barriers (Meldrum, 1990).

How Did Unspoken Thoughts and Assumptions
Affect the Interaction?

   From Louise's unspoken thoughts we can infer that she was trying to be as conscientious as possible; however, there are a lot of basic questions that we must ask ourselves when dealing with dementia patients and Louise seems to assume that she has things "under control." There is an additional mental checklist that Louise needs to think through to evaluate the customer: Is there an impaired level of consciousness or does she look sleepy? Is she making direct eye contact, thereby seeming to *try* her best to communicate? Does she seem to tire easily from such a short conversation? Does her speech sound normal or is it filled with long pauses? Does she appear to be having hearing difficulties? Louise's instincts to observe closely and follow up carefully were absolutely correct, but she did not gather enough information to better assess Mrs. O'Clair's condition.

How Did the Communication Strategies Affect the Outcome?

It is easy to become impatient with older customers who seem slow to "catch on." Many retail pharmacists develop a real "attitude" toward elderly customers with multiple mental and physical health problems. Louise did manage to give Mrs. O'Clair "minimal empathy" by acknowledging that it is scary to get lost and end up in the pharmacy without being fully conscious of it. Also, she was very specific with the customer about how she was going to write out the directions.

But Louise did not verify the patient's understanding out loud. Before trying to instruct the patient, the pharmacist should have verified that Mrs. O'Clair could state back her proper address. In fact, the overall communication difficulty in the interaction is that the pharmacist did too much talking and not enough questioning. Louise is busy writing out directions before she ascertains whether or not Mrs. O'Clair can read. Still, Louise does do a good job of explaining why she would like to send the woman home with a timer system and how the family members could be brought into the patient care plan.

How Could This Have Been Handled Differently?

There are a few additional things a pharmacist can do to better interact with patients with organic mental health problems. These patients should be continued to be addressed by their full names in a slower-than-average speed voice. The pharmacist should find ways to reinforce who they are, what they are dispensing, and reasons for compliance. Do not hurry dementia patients, because although their attention span is short they can comprehend well at times. Pharmacists should make sure they are positioned directly in the patient's line of vision so that they can pick up more about the consultation. The pharmacist should write down his or her own name and the pharmacy's name for the customers to take away with them. In brief, Louise did take some effective action with Mrs. O'Clair and just needs to be a bit more sensitive to the specialized needs of individuals with this type of condition.

"HOW LONG IS THAT ANTIBIOTIC SUPPOSED TO LAST US?"

Background

A regular customer enters the store, picks up some cough and cold O.T.C.s, and comes to the bench to get his daughter's Amoxicillin prescription. Alice dispenses the medication.

[Alice's unspoken thoughts are italicized and set off by brackets.]

Mr. Solomon: "How long is this antibiotic supposed to last us?" (Customer has obvious cold symptoms.)

Alice: [*Is he leading up to something?*] "This is a standard ten-day dose."

Mr. Solomon: "You know, this is the third time my daughter has gotten this in the last three months and she isn't feeling any better."

Alice: [*He sounds agitated.*] "Do you give it to her continually until the bottle is empty?"

Mr. Solomon: "Yes, but there is never ten days worth of medicine in that bottle. Maybe you folks don't put enough in."

Alice: "Do you read the directions on the bottle for reconstitution? Are you using a proper measuring spoon, not a kitchen teaspoon?" [*I wonder if he feels like I'm insulting his intelligence.*]

Mr. Solomon: "I use a kitchen spoon but that shouldn't make that much of a difference. I keep paying 46 dollars for nothing."

Alice: "Perhaps you should get in touch with your doctor and try something else."

Mr. Solomon: "I guess so."

Case Commentary

What Happened?

This was not the most helpful conversation in the history of pharmacist-patient counseling. The customer is picking up his third prescription for his daughter and he is getting very frustrated that the previous prescriptions haven't worked. Instead of empathizing with Mr. Solomon's situation, Alice "quizzed" him pretty extensively. When people are "quizzed," they often feel as if they are being needlessly interrogated and led.

How Did Unspoken Thoughts and Assumptions Affect the Interaction?

As soon as Mr. Solomon began to ask Alice about the length of treatment, she felt that "something was up." In her unspoken thoughts she was aware that he was agitated, and yet she didn't say anything to acknowledge his state of mind. Alice is actively wondering whether or not she is being effective and yet she doesn't surface this doubt to him nor does she manage to change her approach mid-conversation. Why is it that we can have many "clues" going off in our head and still not respond effectively? How is it that we cannot seem to use the very accurate perceptions that we may hold?

How Did the Communication Strategies Affect the Outcome?

Alice's side of the conversation ranged from statements of the obvious ("Perhaps you should get in touch with your doctor . . . ") to somewhat insulting questions ("Did you read the directions?"). Mr.

Solomon would feel like an idiot should he answer one of Alice's questions "incorrectly" (e.g., "Do you give it to her continually until the bottle is empty?"). This is a good example of how a seemingly simple, insignificant case of a common refill can nevertheless be mishandled to such an extent that no real communication takes place.

How Could This Have Been Handled Differently?

Instead of asking a series of loaded, leading, closed-ended questions, Alice should have asked Mr. Solomon some open-ended questions that at least wouldn't have seemed insulting. "How do you give the medication?" would have been a good place to start. She also could have said something like: "After three trips down here and paying for a new refill each time, you must be pretty tired of this," or "I'll bet you're getting a little more worried about your daughter each time it fails to clear up." Alice never really addresses Mr. Solomon's concerns about being ripped off, perhaps by saying something like: "Sounds like you're concerned that we double-check the amount of the medication before dispensing it to you and I can assure you that we do just that," or "I'm wondering what it is that we can do or say to help you today?" The upset customer always wants to feel heard, and it is in the best interest of the pharmacist to give them that respect.

"YOU DIDN'T TELL ME I COULDN'T HAVE A DRINK"

Background

It is a hot Friday night 15 minutes before a small pharmacy is scheduled to close. Jim the pharmacist is tired and wants to go home. Mr. Capano comes in holding an ice pack on his mouth. He has obviously just had extensive dental work.

[Jim's unspoken thoughts are italicized and set off by brackets.]

Jim: [*Great, we'll never get out of here on time.*] "What can we do for you tonight?"

Mr. Capano: "Can you fill this for me quick?" (Shaky voice.)

Jim: [*He looks bad.*] "That will be about ten minutes."

Mr. Capano: "Please hurry, I'm in pain."

Jim: "Right away." (Five minutes pass.) "O.K., did the doctor tell you how to take this?" [*Please say yes.*]

Mr. Capano: "I guess so."

Jim: [*I'm outta here.*] "O.K. then, thanks and have a good night."

(The next day.)

Mr. Capano: "Young man, you gave me these pills last night and you didn't tell me I couldn't have a drink. I got a terrible headache and felt sick on top of the pain from my teeth."

Jim: [*Can't he read?*] "The vial had a red sticker on it telling you not to use alcohol with it."

Mr. Capano: "I was in pain; I didn't have time to read a little sticker."

Jim: [*Guess I have to sound sorry.*] "I'm sorry that it caused you pain."

Mr. Capano: "In the future please treat your customers like human beings."

Jim: [*I'm glad he's leaving.*] "Sorry for the inconvenience."

Mr. Capano: "I have nothing else to say, so goodbye."

Jim: "Sorry for the misunderstanding. Have a good day."

Case Commentary

What Happened?

It seems that Jim had his mind more on when he was getting out of work than on how to be most helpful to his customer. Unfortunately, it is not uncommon for customers to lose their right to education and care when pharmacists cannot get beyond their own concerns of the moment. The rush job that Mr. Capano got was ultimately to cost Jim more time in the end. Not only did he have to deal with Mr. Capano a second time, but he will now have to spend time worrying about his liability in the situation.

How Did Unspoken Thoughts and Assumptions Affect the Interaction?

Jim's unspoken thoughts show a constant focus on getting rid of the customer. He shows a sign of listening with his eyes ("He looks bad"), but he does not use this information to help him deal with Mr. Capano. He thinks "Please say yes" about the doctor having given instructions on how to take the medication, and he is trying to push the customer into agreement for the sake of expedience. There is a tone of disparagement when he thinks "Can't he read?" If he is in fact illiterate, it is nothing to feel superior about. By the time Jim thinks "Guess I'll have to sound sorry," his sincerity is more than suspect. It is amazing how often a realistic fear (getting sued because of failure to counsel) results in anger toward the customer.

How Did the Communication Strategies Affect the Outcome?

It is easy to see that the problem with the initial interaction was the all too common problem of the closed, leading question. When Mr. Capano came in the next day to complain about the discomfort that he had to go through, he was rewarded with a condescending slap on the wrist ("The vial had a sticker on it telling you not to . . ."). After this initial response, Jim kept on trying to appease Mr. Capano by saying he was "sorry." Mr. Capano expressed that he felt that his very "personhood" was mistreated to which Jim responded "Sorry for the inconvenience." All of Jim's "sorrys" sounded empty, bogus, mindless, and automatic. Anyone can say sorry in a thoughtless, perfunctory fashion and it never communicates empathy, let alone a bare minimum of real sympathy. The overuse of sorry means the word loses its value and offers no comfort at all to a troubled customer or co-worker. Jim's series of "sorrys" obviously had no effect on Mr. Capano who ended the interaction while he was still upset.

How Could This Have Been Handled Differently?

Obviously Jim needed to verify Mr. Capano's understanding and when he came back the next day Jim needed to refrain from trying to shift the blame completely away from himself. A reflective response would have been more appropriate: "Sounds like you're upset because you wanted me to give you more information on side effects," to which Mr. Capano would have probably said something like "Damn right you should have!" Jim should then have come back with "So you had to put up with a terrible headache that could have been completely avoided." By showing Mr. Capano that he "gets it," Jim will create more of a bond between them that may restore some of the lost trust. It doesn't hurt to remind ourselves that practitioners with good human relations skills are rarely the ones who get sued or reported to their superiors. Additionally, by employing these skills we can get beyond the level of personal interest, and create more fair conditions for both parties in the interpersonal dialogue.

Chapter 4

Conflict with Co-Workers in the Community Pharmacy

"I'M JUST DOING MY JOB HERE"

Background

Amy is the daughter of the owner/manager of Ned's Pharmacy. She has been working in the business for years as a manager and is herself a fifth-year pharmacy student. It is the last few hours of a long day and Amy and Jane (the full-time pharmacist) are the only employees left in the store. Both women are approximately the same age and generally work closely together. Amy had hired Jane years ago and Jane had proven that she could run an efficient Rx counter.

[Amy's unspoken thoughts are italicized and set off by brackets.]

Amy: "Can you help me tonight with some O.T.C. inventory and unpacking some boxes?"

Jane: "I'm busy now, but I'll see what I can get done after I finish here."

Amy: [*She's trying to blow me off.*] "Are you filling scripts, or are you just catching up on profiles?"

Jane: "Why do you ask?"

Amy: [*No sense hinting around.*] "I have to get this inventory done. I can't do it all by myself and the pharmacist in a small store should not consider any one part of the business more important than another."

Jane: "I'd be happy to help you as soon as I'm finished with my patient profiles."

Amy: "Look, not having the profiles totally up-to-date isn't as important as getting inventory done."

Jane: "If you would stop starting so many projects and start finishing up some you wouldn't be so far behind."

Amy: [*I handle all your overflow of customers.*] "I'm behind because I have to wait on customers, and answer your questions, and since you've never done my job, how would you know?"

Jane: "It just seems like you're fine and easy to work with, then all of a sudden you're nervous about a deadline. You're not very consistent."

Amy: [*I'll bet she resents me.*] "Maybe so, and I'm sorry, but I'll tell you something; you are always undermining my decisions and underestimating everyone's ability. You check up on other people and put your two cents in. But if I take an initiative you decide it's not important and don't cooperate."

Jane: "Sometimes I feel as if you take out your personal problems on me."

Amy: "I hope that isn't true. There really isn't anything bothering me."

Case Commentary

What Happened?

Amy had high hopes of getting a lot accomplished with the help of her co-worker but it certainly didn't turn out that way. Although Amy did not intend to, she communicated to Jane that her work wasn't that important in comparison to Amy's obsession about her own. Amy further communicates that she is somewhat insulted that Jane is rather unsympathetic. When we examine the progression of the dialogue, both seem to be saying, "So you think you have it tough! Look at all I do!" No one likes the job of unpacking and reordering inventory and yet the resistance to the task that was hanging heavily in the air was never discussed explicitly. The bad feeling created here will no doubt affect the next conversation they have. Perhaps both will adopt the common avoidance style as they return to their separate corners to wait for things to blow over, and yet there are very few interpersonal problems that the passage of time alone will resolve.

How Did Unspoken Thoughts and Assumptions Affect the Interaction?

From the very beginning, Amy assumes the worst about Jane's intentions. She believes that Jane is deliberately and consciously scheming to get out of helping her. Obviously this attitude would affect her choice of words and approach to Jane. Amy believes that Jane will refuse to take a hint "Because she doesn't want to help." By the end of the dialogue, Amy believes that not only doesn't Jane want to help with non-pharmacy-related tasks, but that she will resist everything that Amy suggests, simply for the sake of being insubordinate. Amy is operating on an unspoken "You scratch my back and I'll scratch yours" mentality. She wants Jane to recognize that because she helps Jane with customers, helping her with non-pharmacy business is only fair. Jane may or may not see this as an even exchange and Amy doesn't encourage an open discussion of the issue.

How Did the Communication Strategies Affect the Outcome?

Amy wanted to communicate that in the small independent pharmacy, the pharmacist is also a business employee. The way that Amy constructs her first question is pure entrapment. "Are you filling scripts or are you just catching up on profiles?" This type of leading, closed question is obviously communicating that the asker has predetermined which activity is important and which isn't. No one likes to be told what part of their job function is worthy. We want to decide that for ourselves. Imagine saying to a lawyer friend: "Are you in court today, or are you just meeting with clients?" We will vigorously defend that part of our job that is being devalued.

Although Amy has just communicated that she is the judge of

what is a priority, she goes on to announce that all things are equal: "The pharmacist should not consider any one part of the business more important than another." Mixed messages like this are very irritating for the receiver.

Amy continuously tries to 'counter-argue' Jane's statements about finishing the profiles. When Jane realizes that the broken record response is not going to work, she begins to attack on a more personal level. Within seconds, the focus of the discussion leaves the task at hand and begins to focus on what is wrong with each person's personality. Each seems to imply that she is the only one who really works diligently. Neither woman is willing to take no for an answer so both end up looking insanely demanding in the eyes of the other. Although their past history of working together included a lot of mutual respect, none of it comes through in this exchange.

How Could This Have Been Handled Differently?

Amy's objective was to get support for her inventory work and her fear was that Jane would resent her style of soliciting that help. She didn't get the help she needed and we can safely infer that Jane resented her approach. Like most of us, Amy created a situation that she hates. And like all of us, there are other more effective communication options available to her.

Amy could have said one or several of the following statements: "I can see that you're working on the computerized profiles and that's important, but I'm in a bit of a bind and I was hoping to recruit you to help me . . . I'm uncomfortable when I feel that I have to put on my Manager's hat to make a request that we work on a project because I'm always afraid that I'll be resented. I realize that by asking you at the last minute it seems like I'm saying that my work is more important than yours; I hope you know I respect your professionalism and will try to continue to help you when you're under pressure . . . I realize that it's a pattern for me to be running behind on inventory projects and deadlines and I'm not sure how much of it is because of not employing enough clerks . . . If we work together on this project tonight, can we also brainstorm on how to avoid these deadlocks in the future? . . . I'd like to hear your ideas because I don't think I can come up with a fair answer alone."

If Amy persists in using open, collaborative communication that takes ownership for her contribution to the problem and avoids blaming others, she can expect all of the pharmacy's employees to react more favorably toward her.

"ACCIDENTS HAPPEN"

Background

Mary works at Instant-Care Pharmacy, a large home health care pharmacy that employs approximately 200 people. There is a separate part of the pharmacy that deals directly in the distribution of "easy access" medication. Steven, the nephew of the owner of Instant-Care, is employed in the easy access department. While filling a prescription for a patient, Mary noticed a shortage of Dilantin and went to get more. She asked Steven to direct her to where the drug was kept and as she opened the jar a few capsules broke in her hand. Dilantin is irritating to the nose, eyes, and throat if the powder is released. Steven reacted strongly to the accident.

[Mary's unspoken thoughts are italicized and set off by brackets.]

Mary: "Is there any Dilantin back here?"

Steven: "Yup, third shelf."

Mary: "Do you have a paper towel? A capsule just broke in my hand."

Steven: "What? Are you an idiot? That stuff makes my nose water and throat hurt. Clean it up!"

Mary: [*He looks like he's having a heart attack, but it's nowhere near him. What a crybaby; I'm the one inhaling the fumes. Why does he have to be the owner's nephew?*] "Steven, accidents happen."

Steven: "I don't care how it happened, obviously you're not careful enough. Where did you go to school anyway?"

Mary: [*You're lucky I catch your drug errors all the time.*] "Steven, you're not even near it. I'll clean it up right away–this isn't a disaster, you know."

Steven: "I can't believe you!"

Mary: [*He's so cranky!*] "O.K. Steven, don't push me! Drop the subject or you won't like it. I guarantee it."

Steven: "I won't drop it. I can't believe you did this."

Mary: [*How would you like a gram of Dilantin powder up your nose?*] "Steven, I'm sick of your crap. Get off my back before I really lose my temper and start throwing things–starting with this Dilantin bottle."

(Mary stomps off, leaving mess behind.)

Case Commentary

What Happened?

This screaming match picked up heat very quickly. In the high volume, high stress atmosphere of the pharmacy, it is not unusual to witness tempers flaring. As each person got angrier, more emotionally charged words were exchanged. Yet, often when there is anger there is a fear that triggers such strong reactions. Mary was later to learn that Steven is highly allergic to many chemicals and had reacted initially out of deep concern for his own well-being.

How Did Unspoken Thoughts and Assumptions
Affect the Interaction?

One of Mary's first unspoken observations was that Steven looked ill–like he was having a coronary. That was a clue to the seriousness of the situation for him, and yet she did not address this aloud. Often we need to listen with our eyes as well as with our ears. Mary seems to assume that because Steven is related to the owner he is taking special liberties with verbal abuse. Perhaps the assumption lessens her empathy and compassion for his obvious distress.

Mary's unspoken thoughts make it clear that she has little respect for Steven because he makes prescription mistakes, which to her seems to be another reason to dismiss him as a crank. Mary's unspoken assumptions about Steven keep her from wondering *why* Steven is so upset. She is sure she *knows* why–he's an unreasonable, cranky, spoiled, nepotistic blunderer. Mary believes that a good co-worker would accept that "accidents happen" and drop it. Why doesn't she ask herself why he is not able to let it go easily, and then be *genuinely* curious about the answer (instead of looking for more evidence of his personality defects).

How Did the Communication Strategies Affect the Outcome?

Mary's main behavioral strategy was to try to convince Steven that the accident was no big deal. He said it was. She said it wasn't. Ad nauseam. It reminds us of playground dynamics among five-year-olds. "I'm right." "No! I'm right!" Our language is a bit more sophisticated in adulthood, but the results are not any better. Somebody still gets punched, runs away, or "tells."

When a communication strategy does not seem to be working for us, why is it that we cannot seem to try something new or different? These chronic conflict situations so often seem to operate like games of "Bluff Poker." Instead of playing hands we play with verbal abuse chips (e.g., "Where did you go to school anyway?) Automatically and without thinking we say "O.K., I'll match those verbal abuse chips and I'll raise you ten" (e.g., "I'm sick of your crap."). We learned this game in the playground and we cannot seem to appreciate that in games of competitive strategy, both people eventually get hurt.

How Could This Have Been Handled Differently?

A quick fix solution might have Mary asking Steven to leave the room for a moment while she cleaned up. This would relieve the anxiety he felt about his health and prove that Mary took him seriously enough to take immediate action.

Early on in the dialogue, Mary needed to show Steven that she saw and heard the extent of his panic. A simple statement like, "I can see that you're upset" might have brought forth more needed information: "Damn right I'm upset. I'm allergic as hell to that stuff!" By immediately trying to defend herself, Mary missed her opportunity to find out the real problem.

There is a real qualitative difference between demanding that someone "drop it" and finding out why they don't seem to be able to. Mary needed to stop the vicious back and forth cycle with a comment like "I've heard you criticize me three times now for being careless, and I've heard myself try to explain three times that it was an accident. How is it that we don't seem to be able to come to an understanding together?" This open-ended question takes the focus off the broken record aspects of the "content" of the problem (the ramifications of the accident) and puts the focus on the "process" of the interaction between the parties in conflict. Stopping to ask ourselves why we cannot negotiate a conflict successfully today will give us knowledge to better manage our conflicts of tomorrow.

"I'M TRYING TO BE REASONABLE"

Background

Jim had been working part time for four months in a very large store which was a branch of National Name Chain Stores Inc. One supervisor was in charge of scheduling workers in several of the stores in the urban area. Upon taking on this second job, Jim thought he had been very clear that his availability was limited to Mondays, Thursday evenings, and Saturday mornings. Jim reported for work as usual on the Monday before the Fourth of July.

[Jim's unspoken thoughts are italicized and set off by brackets.]

Jim: "I have just come all the way down here to work tonight only to be told I was not on tonight. What's going on?"

Dir. of Scheduling: (reached by phone) "Hang on a minute please . . . you will be working tomorrow night."

Jim: [*That's it? No explanation?*] "That cannot be. I have specifically informed you that I am only free to work on Mondays, Thursdays, and Saturdays."

Dir. of Scheduling: "Look, the work schedule has been up for two weeks already; you should have known that you were working tomorrow night."

Jim: [*He's showing his true colors.*] "That is beside the point. I have stated clearly that I could work only on those days I asked for."

Dir. of Scheduling: "It is your responsibility to check the work schedule. Besides, I asked you before about working holidays and you said O.K."

Jim: [*We're going in circles here. Now he's lying.*] "I never talked to you about that. I've only spoken to you once and that was to tell you the times I was free to work."

Dir. of Scheduling: (In a sarcastic tone.) "So you're saying I have to spoil my own plans and find someone to replace you or to work myself, right?"

Jim: [*He's so unreasonable. We're both so upset.*] "I am trying to be reasonable here and I'd appreciate it if you'd do likewise."

Dir. of Scheduling: "You'd better talk to your manager about this one."

Jim: "You bet I will." [*I'm going to tell her how awful you are.*]

Case Commentary

What Happened?

Jim probably entered this conversation with the straightforward goal of finding out why he was scheduled for a Tuesday when he thought he specified that he could not come in on Tuesdays. He didn't think this was going to be a "big deal" and his next day holiday plans figured prominently in his mind. Both people fell into the all too familiar trap of conflict escalation described in Chapter One. Instead of repeatedly telling the scheduling officer that he was wrong, Jim could have appealed for help in clarifying what was going on and how the mistake had happened. If in fact the Director of Scheduling was consciously aware that he had made a mistake, there is almost zero probability that he will admit it at this point. "Saving face" seems so vitally important in the midst of a battle. What people don't seem to appreciate is that even if one "wins" a battle like this one, the war will still rage on through long-term strategies of retaliation. Most likely, Jim's and the Director of Scheduling's superiors and subordinates will all hear about this one and the negative impressions formed of Jim and the Director may affect many of their interactions for months or years to come.

How Did Unspoken Thoughts and Assumptions Affect the Interaction?

Jim seems to conclude that the scheduling director is deliberately abusing his authority. His unspoken thoughts seem to indicate resentment of their status differences (e.g., "That's it, no explanations?"). When the Director of Scheduling became exasperated and lapsed into blaming language ("You should have known"), Jim sees it as a moment of authenticity ("true colors") rather than the by-product of stress and burnout. You can bet that Jim's explanations for his own blaming strategies would sound more generous, compassionate, and of course, "plausible." Jim not only thinks the Director is unreasonable, he believes him to be a liar, an attitude sure to contaminate their future discussions. Jim seems to assume that the Director of Scheduling has *deliberately* failed to acknowledge his request and further enjoys pushing around the part-time "peon" pharmacist.

How Did the Communication Strategies Affect the Outcome?

As we often see in conflicts, Jim has taken the "I'll just stick to my guns and try to wear my opponent down" approach. His opponent responds in kind. The discussion escalates very quickly to a level of personal insult and repeated attempts to fix the blame. Each side tries to end the encounter with the last blow delivered. They both seem to be speaking in pseudo-logic: e.g., "Here is the reason why you are wrong. . . ." The Director of Scheduling attempted to make Jim feel guilty but he was met with a familiar "You're pathetic" comeback. And, of course, both end the encounter with the predictable, thinly veiled threats of retaliation. Isn't it funny how as "grown-up" professionals we still haven't gotten beyond "I'm telling my Daddy on you" and "Oh yeah, well my Daddy's bigger than yours."

How Could This Have Been Handled Differently?

When people take a collaborative approach to communication with colleagues there is only *one* thing they know for certain. They know that they don't know everything there is to know about the situation at hand. They believe that each party involved in the conflict has a piece of the truth and only through patient, non-defensive brainstorming will these pieces be found and put together to form a whole.

Looking back at this situation, what might have happened if Jim admitted at the beginning that he should have checked the work schedule, instead of assuming that it was business as usual during a holiday week? He would have been alerted to a possible conflict well before the fact and constructive action might have been taken. If a non-defensive atmosphere was maintained by both, the Director of Scheduling might have felt free to say that he had forgotten or didn't write down what Jim had said about availability. Had Jim ever taken the time to double-check to see if the message sent was the message heard? There have been national tragedies on airport runways because of simple miscommunications between control towers and pilots. If the two colleagues could come to an agreement that communication had broken down, perhaps they could move on to creative problem-solving instead of fault-finding. Both parties might have been able to come up with ideas about how to get a replacement for Jim.

What was it that prevented Jim from saying what he was thinking ("We are going around in circles")? Often taking the action of pointing out what is really happening calls the game. Simply saying "We are going around in circles" might inspire a different reaction such as "All right, let's stop it." Another way to end the game is to acknowledge the truth, e.g., "I can hear that we are both getting pretty worked up about this." The hallmark of a collaborative communicator lies in one's ability to take what is in the back of one's mind (unspoken thoughts) and say it effectively so that it makes a crucial difference in the destiny of one's relationships. Obviously, Jim could say something like, "I think you're lying to save face," or he could say, "It seems that what you understand to be true and what I understand to be true are two totally different things; where do we go from here?" By employing collaborative strategies, we build relationships that are strong and productive, not brittle and negative.

"THANKS FOR WORKING WITH ME ON THIS"

Background

Sally, a pharmacy student, has been working in the same pharmacy for over two years. It is a large volume operation and requires many employees to run. The majority of employees are students and scheduling is a major issue. All switches in schedule after posting have to be approved by a supervisor. Since the pharmacy is open 365 days a year and for 14 hours a day, students are often required to work nights, holidays, and weekends. Sally had worked some rough understaffed shifts lately and was feeling a little burnt out. Recently, Sally's hours were rearranged against her preferences and she was considering quitting or at least making her unhappiness known. She arranges to meet privately with her manager to discuss hours and her concerns about pharmacy obligations.

[Sally's unspoken thoughts are italicized and set off by brackets.]

Manager: "Sally, let's have that talk you asked about; we can go into Tom's office where it's quiet."

Sally: [*I want to get things out in the open,*] "Great! I've been wanting to talk but if it's too busy I can come in tomorrow." [*Why did I say that–what an ingrained reflex.*]

Manager: "No, I have my wife doing the pick-up at Day Care so I could stay late and talk with you."

Sally: [*He went to a lot of trouble.*] "Thanks, I appreciate your efforts. Before we begin, I hope you don't think I'm planning to quit."

Manager: "I didn't think it was that bad, but I picked up that some things are bothering you."

Sally: [*News travels fast. I'm glad I didn't put off talking with him.*] "I feel that I have been treated fairly with respect to scheduling until recently. In the past I've been accommodating and also helped out by working extra hours during the holidays and when we were short-handed." [*I only took one day for Thanksgiving and two for Christmas and I live out of state.*]

Manager: "You've always been great about that."

Sally: "Well, lately I've had problems on days I requested off and I don't understand why. Plus my Tuesday hours got cut. I'm worried that because I'm a senior you're trying to phase me out a bit at a time."

Manager: "Oh, not at all. We depend on you so much, sometimes to the point of taking advantage of you to fill in extra hours. You're the first person I think of to put new students with–it's just that you never voice your concerns about these things."

Sally: [*I've never felt this valuable before.*] "I realize that, which is why I wanted to talk to you about my future here."

Manager: "Do you plan on staying on after the Boards?"

Sally: "Yes, but I need more weekends off to rest and prepare for the Boards."

Manager: "I'm glad you're thinking about this now."

Sally: [*He seems to understand where I'm coming from.*] "Well, I really want to work with you in coming up with a schedule that's fair to both of us."

Manager: "Come up with a temporary three-month schedule and we'll talk again."

Sally: "Thanks for talking with me. I feel better."

Case Commentary

What Happened?

Anyone who has worked in a pharmacy knows that the issue of scheduling is always a touchy and potentially volatile one (see previous case). It seems that more often than not, tempers flare and conflict escalates. Yet in this situation, all the crisis, tension, and bad feelings were avoided. So why include this case study in the chapter on conflict with co-workers? It illustrates what can happen when people collaborate and are direct about their wants and needs, while at the same time showing an equal amount of concern for the other party.

Clearly, Sally's discussion with her supervisor was a very big step for her. It is always tempting to avoid potentially tense situations and hope they go away. The issue of scheduling is a major stressor in the lives of both employee and employer. By finding effective ways to deal with the problem directly we save wear and tear on our psyches.

How Did Unspoken Thoughts and Assumptions Affect the Interaction?

One of the joys of collaborative communication is that in learning to say what you think more effectively, you waste less energy on untested assumptions about what the other person is thinking. Notice how Sally's unspoken thoughts are fairly straightforward and unsuspicious, in contrast to the thinking of the other characters in cases in this chapter. For example, Sally had the suspicion that management might be trying to phase her out before she passed the Boards (and required a raise). People with a competitive style of conflict management would avoid saying this aloud at all costs. After all, if there was any truth to it, it would be a big blow to the ego and very difficult to save face.

It is very liberating to be able to say what you fear instead of reacting to it or trying to compensate for it. For example, Sally was afraid that her manager would think she had arranged the meeting to threaten to quit, so she eliminated that fear right away by addressing it. So often we have interactions and we fume to ourselves, "I just know he thinks I'm lying to him . . . or trying to humor him . . . or trying to console him . . ." and so on, but we never seem to say these fears aloud.

This is similar to the case of the college professor who, upon seeing a few sleeping heads among many, decides that the class thinks she's boring and therefore tries to speed up her rate of speaking to minimize the damage. She starts speaking in a manic, nervous way and becomes less comprehensible and as a result, more and more students mentally wander off into never-never land. She has created more of what she hates. What stops her from saying "I see a few nodding heads out there and I'm wondering if it's me or if it's Senior Week hangover. If it is my approach to the material, can you help me out with some ideas about how you can best learn this?" But instead our professor will probably just let the class go early for the tenth time this semester. It is very hard to break away from the behavior that so many have modeled for us.

How Did the Communication Strategies Affect the Outcome?

Sally has many strengths to comment on. First, Sally seems to appreciate the value of being specific. Instead of implying that she has been treated shabbily for an indefinite period she comes right to the point with specific examples of her problem with scheduling changes. She communicates her intention to be reasonable and to take the Manager's difficulties into account. She avoids sarcasm and comes across as confident and self-assured. Sally verbalizes her appreciation of her manager's efforts and lets him know she feels good about their relationship. All of this effort towards effective communication will pay off the next time she and her boss need to talk about a problem, a pay raise, or a promotion. Whereas in previous cases we witnessed a process of hostile interpersonal "Bluff Poker" with a growing pile of verbal aggression chips being tossed in from both sides, in this case as each side offers a reasonable empathic statement the other responds in kind.

How Could This Have Been Handled Differently?

There is not much to say here because both people seemed to put forth a worthy effort. Sally almost "chickened out" in the beginning when she was tempted to return to her old pattern of avoidance. She seems to have achieved her objectives of communicating how she felt about unexplained changes in the schedule and her thoughts on her future with this pharmacy.

"YOU CAN'T FIRE ME BECAUSE I QUIT"

Background

Andy has been working for four years at the Smithville branch of Small Chain Drug, Inc. Because of his loyal service, he was promoted to manager at the new store in Jonesville. Andy was an excellent assistant manager at Smithville and things have not been running smoothly there since he left. The Assistant Supervisor of Personnel for Small Chain Drug, Inc. calls with a request.

[Andy's unspoken thoughts are italicized and set off by brackets.]

Asst. Super.: "Hi Andy, it's Sue. How are you?"

Andy: "Hi, what's up?" [*What the hell does she want?*]

Asst. Super.: "Well, I want to know if you'll work in Smithville two days a week to help out."

Andy: "I left for this promotion and I don't want to go back." [*If she did her job right she wouldn't have to ask me.*]

Asst. Super.: "Please, I'd really appreciate it. I know you just didn't like it because it wasn't your store."

Andy: "This is where I belong and they need me here too. How can you expect me to go back where I just came from?"

Asst. Super.: "It's just helping out. I really need your help. Won't you do it?"

Andy: "Well, okay, but just for two weeks, maximum." [*I'm sick of her whining, I wish she would leave me alone. What a sap I am.*]

Asst. Super.: "Thanks a lot."

(Two weeks later a call comes from the head of Personnel for Small Chain Drugs, Inc.)

Dir. Personnel: "Hi Andy. How are you? I understand that you left Smithville and that you did so through your own decision."

Andy: [*Why is he calling me? What's he got to do with this? What is going on here?*] "Yeah, I did. I had told your assistant that I was going to go back in two weeks. I told the folks at Smithville that Friday would be my last day and that I would be coming back here to Jonesville."

Dir. Personnel: "Well I don't know why you were there and who put you there but we cannot have pharmacists making these kinds of decisions by themselves."

Andy: [*What is he talking about? What decisions? This idiot believes anything anyone tells him. What a jerk.*] "What decisions? You mean I cannot run my own life? I told your assistant when I would leave and she said fine. If she would just do her job in the first place we wouldn't be having these problems. I'm just trying to do my job."

Dir. Personnel: "Well we can't and won't have this."

Andy: [*I don't believe this is happening, all because I try to do someone a favor. Why me?*] "What is going on, why is this such a big deal? If you want my two week notice, you've got it."

Dir. Personnel: "I don't think you have two weeks."

Andy: [*You can't have the last word. I can't believe what I'm saying.*] "Oh, I see, just like that after four years of loyal service. God, I've only called in sick four days in four years and I've done everyone in this company a favor, including you. Now it doesn't matter, you can't fire me 'cause I quit. You are all a bunch of losers."

Case Commentary

What Happened?

A long-term employee was lost unnecessarily. A well-earned promotion to management went down the drain. Why? Both parties' defenses were triggered and they quickly escalated to the point of difficult return. (Hopefully there is no such thing as a point of no return.) A competitive "fight to win" mentality overcame both Andy and the Director of Personnel and neither stepped back to examine the situation they had created.

It would be easy to reach the conclusion that Andy simply should never do anyone favors if it's at his own expense. However, it was not so much of a problem that the favor itself was granted. It was a failure to communicate carefully about the terms of the favor. Andy never checked in with the Assistant to see if his two-week maximum was both heard and agreed with. Andy wanted to make the point that his old store was not his responsibility anymore. Why couldn't he find an effective way to get that message across?

How Did Unspoken Thoughts and Assumptions Affect the Interaction?

Andy was very shocked that the Director of Personnel called him. It seems he thought that if the Assistant Supervisor had a problem with him she would confront him directly. From the very start, Andy believed that the Assistant Supervisor was incompetent. If he believed her to be incompetent, why didn't he help her to do her job or at the very least prove that he had made a responsible decision in returning to Smithville?

It seems that Andy's silent reasoning went something like this: "I think the Assistant Supervisor is too incompetent to place an effective person in my old job at Smithville. In two weeks time I'll have more proof that I'm right because she still won't have brought in someone new. God knows I'm not going to help her or try to find out and understand her difficulties. It's not my job. Two weeks will pass and she'll be stuck, ha! Oh well, at least I told her that soon she won't be able to use me to buy time."

If Andy holds this negative view of the Assistant Supervisor, there is no doubt his tone of voice and word choice communicates his opinion to her very directly. And yet, on some level he still expects her to keep talking to him about staffing problems. Similarly, Andy seems to see the Director of Personnel as an unthinking spokesperson for his assistant. Andy wonders why the person believes the assistant's side of the story without asking him about it.

How Did the Communication Strategies Affect the Outcome?

Andy seemed to believe it was important to maintain strength in his position and "not back down." He also spent a lot of time blaming the assistant, which probably didn't endear him to the

Director. Neither Andy nor the Director presented the facts of the situation as they had originally perceived them. The strategy of quitting before being fired is always a desperate grasp at dignity. "Gunny-sacking" the company as a whole as Andy did in the end is not exactly feedback that will be acted upon to improve management practices. The ramifications of this misunderstanding were terribly unfortunate.

How Could This Have Been Handled Differently?

At the point that Andy decided to grant the favor of working back at Smithville he could have said: "Although I would rather stay full time at my current position, I will help you for two weeks to give you some time to find a replacement. However, I'm worried that in two weeks time we will still be in the same position. Is there anything that I can do or advice I can offer to facilitate this transition?" Can you please call me a few times over the next two weeks so I can be assured that the hiring process is still on track?"

Later, the Director "accused" Andy of making unilateral decisions and this was a good opportunity for Andy to "check in" with what he was hearing. "Sounds like you think I'm authorizing myself to switch stores without making an explicit agreement with your assistant. I thought I did have an explicit agreement with her. Perhaps I wasn't as clear as possible and we misunderstood each other." This is a great improvement over attacking the Director's assistant. If the Director persists in an accusatory tone, Andy can say: "I'm certainly confused here, I've acted in ways I've thought were proper and authorized (re-explains his side of the story), and yet I get the feeling that I've got a 'reputation' that is undeserved." Also, Andy needed to pick up on and respond to the Director's statement: "I don't know why you were there or who put you there, I really don't know anything about this. . . ." This was Andy's cue to start explaining, rather than defending and blaming.

PART II:
COMMUNICATION
IN THE HOSPITAL PHARMACY

It is quite clear from the previous section on community practice that most of the interpersonal "challenges" take place between the pharmacist and the customer. In hospital practice, some of the most stressful interactions take place between members of the health care team. For example, the author knows of a case where a clinical pharmacist responded to a physician's request for drug information by researching the question for hours in a variety of sources. When she called the doctor back, he said, "Nevermind, I just went with something I saw in the P.D.R." How can the pharmacist keep this situation from being repeated? It is difficult for pharmacists to feel like valued and respected members of the health care team when they are also convinced that the nurses are abusing their S.T.A.T. privileges several times during a single shift. To do effective discharge counseling, pharmacists must plan carefully with these very same nurses who sometimes seem oblivious to what the pharmacist's job actually entails. Nurses often end up doing the patient's outgoing consultation because of a lack of coordination through communication. Maintaining credibility through effective communication is a vitally important element of the hospital pharmacist's job.

Because so many hospitals have outpatient pharmacies that are set up similarly to H.M.O.s and community settings, the reader will find several cases in this section that are quite comparable to situations that arise in retail practice. For instance, excellent questioning skills are essential for clinical pharmacists in conducting effective medical interviews.

Whether communicating with a co-worker or a patient, the hospital pharmacist is most often functioning as an educator. When we think back about the truly great teachers in our lives, it always seems that we learned the most from those who talked with us instead of at us. Educators who take the time to adapt to the individual needs of their students get the best results. When members of the health care team attempt to communicate with each other and their patients, they need to take similar steps to ensure that they are speaking each other's language. In the cases that follow, hospital and H.M.O. pharmacists experience greater and lesser degrees of success with their communicative challenges. Let's take a look at some situations calling for skills in managing conflict with patients, counseling patients, and handling confrontations with co-workers.

Chapter 5

Conflict with Patients in the Hospital Pharmacy

"THE DOCTOR WILL GIVE YOU THE PRESCRIPTION LATER"

Background

It is a hot summer day about an hour before the closing of the outpatient window at the hospital pharmacy. A patient comes in requesting Halcyon with no oral or written prescription. Ed must explain why she can't have the drug.

[Ed's unspoken thoughts are italicized and set off by brackets.]

Ms. Perry: "Hi, I'd like the Halcyon tablet my doctor told me about. I need 30 pills of 0.25 mg, please."

Ed: "OK. Can I have your prescription?"

Ms. Perry: "The doctor will give you the prescription later."

Ed: [*This is a new one.*] "I need a prescription to dispense anything."

Ms. Perry: "No, my doctor said I'm all set and that he'll send you a note after I pick it up."

Ed: [*No way!*] "Maybe you mean he'll call us with the prescription? We haven't heard from him yet."

Ms. Perry: (getting loud) "Listen, he didn't mention an oral prescription; this is how we always do it. Why is it different now?"

Ed: [*She's lying and she thinks I'm totally dumb.*] "The law doesn't allow me to do that. Please call your doctor so he can authorize this."

Ms. Perry: "Why are you giving me such a hard time?"

Ed: [*She's worse than our nurses! Unbelievable!*] "You're wasting your time and mine. Just call him."

Ms. Perry: "I don't want to bother him. Let me talk to your boss."

Case Commentary

What Happened?

Ed needs to give a full explanation about why he can't fill prescriptions without the proper documentation. Ms. Perry can't seem to understand what the problem is and Ed's minimal communication style is not helping to get the message across. It wouldn't be too hard to get a prescription from the doctor by phone, but by the end of the exchange, Ms. Perry is convinced that she has been given a hard time totally needlessly and she has revenge on her mind.

How Did Unspoken Thoughts and Assumptions
Affect the Interaction?

Ed is caught off guard by the request and we can tell from reviewing his unspoken thoughts that he has never had a patient request drugs without a prescription before. Ed also makes a number of very negative assumptions that shape his behavior. He believes that the customer is deliberately lying to him. This may be, but more likely the patient is confused and doesn't realize that when she has picked up prescriptions in the past the doctor has called ahead. Why doesn't Ed allow for this possibility? Instead, Ed reacts as if this woman considers him stupid and is trying to trick him. If Ed continues to believe these things, the chances are slim that he will think of an effective and helpful way of communicating with Ms. Perry.

How Did the Communication Strategies Affect the Outcome?

As a general rule, pharmacists should not send any messages of confirmation before determining if there is going to be a problem with the prescription or not. In many of the cases in this book, the pharmacist's first response to a request is "O.K." and the patient is lead to believe that his or her drugs are forthcoming. Ed persists in putting words in Ms. Perry's mouth without first understanding the cause of her confusion (e.g., "Maybe you mean he'll call us with the prescription?"). The pharmacist jumps right into using the law as a justification for withholding the drug without first explaining why such a policy is needed, which might help Ms. Perry to understand his position. As mentioned in several cases, pharmacists often use the explanation "it's the law" without further elaboration, and patients usually experience that response as robotic and impersonal at best. By the time Ed ends up yelling "You're wasting your time and mine," he has confused and upset the patient to the point that a service complaint will end up in his personnel employment file.

How Could This Have Been Handled Differently?

Ed needed to say more of what was on his mind. For example, from the very beginning he might have said, "I'm a bit confused and surprised; I've never had a patient ask for a drug without a prescription before. Can I ask you a few questions to clarify my confusion?" Ed could then proceed to inquire about how the patient came to believe that there would be no problem obtaining the drug. He also needed to address the patient's mounting frustration, by saying something like: "I can see that you're upset because you didn't think there would be any problem. . . . I'm afraid that a non-negotiable pharmacy law prevents me from dispensing this medication without authorization; it was formulated to keep patients from having easy access to habit-forming or dangerous drugs. Now it's certainly not relevant to you since you've just agreed with your doctor that Halcyon is the best treatment for you, but nevertheless the policy ties my hands in terms of serving you until you or I can reach your doctor." A full and specific detailed explanation often provides the kind of psychological satisfaction the patient is looking for.

"JUST TAKE MY WORD FOR IT"

Background

It is a quiet day in the outpatient pharmacy; Leslie and one pharmacy technician are on duty. There is a question in Leslie's mind of whether a doctor meant to write a prescription for Anusol or Anusol HC. Leslie has been trying to get in touch with the doctor.

[Leslie's unspoken thoughts are italicized and set off by brackets.]

Leslie: "Hi. Can I help you?"

Mr. Audette: "I'd like to pick up the prescription for Audette. It was dropped off this morning."

Leslie: [*I hope he doesn't give me a hard time.*] "I'm sorry, but your prescription isn't ready yet. We need to get in touch with the doctor to find out whether he wants you to have Anusol or Anusol HC, because Anusol is an over-the-counter medication."

Mr. Audette: "I've had HC before; just give me that."

Leslie: [*Here it comes.*] "We don't have any files on that so I can't assume that; I have to verify it."

Mr. Audette: "I'm going on my vacation. Just take my word for it that it was HC. Why would he give me a prescription for an over-the-counter drug?"

Leslie: [*Is he so stupid he thinks I can just give him what he wants? He cares more about his vacation than his prescription.*] "It's not unusual for hospital doctors to write for O.T.C.s."

Mr. Audette: "I'm sure he meant the prescription drug. Now come on, I've got to go."

Leslie: "Then maybe you should have brought the prescription in three days ago when you got it." [*Oops, a bit much, I guess.*]

Mr. Audette: "Don't speak to me that way. Let me speak to your boss."

Leslie: [*So I'm too stupid or something?*] "I'm the boss today, sorry."

Case Commentary

What Happened?

Leslie needed to find out whether or not the patient had taken any type of Anusol in the past and she needed to explain the difference between the types if necessary. She was trying to communicate that the doctor could have been writing for either drug and that her wanting to do the right thing had caused the delay. Unfortunately, Leslie came across as quite unsympathetic to the patient.

How Did Unspoken Thoughts and Assumptions Affect the Interaction?

Leslie thinks to herself, "Is this guy so stupid as to think I can just give him what he wants?" Now, why would this be an issue of stupidity? Isn't this simply an issue of naiveté? Why wouldn't an average patient believe it is O.K. to swap one form of a drug for another? In fact, the public is being educated to believe that it happens all the time with generics. The customer's only "stupidity" is that he is unfamiliar with pharmacy law, but then again, isn't that the pharmacist's job to explain fully? Why act as if the patient is dumb and then hold it against him? Leslie further seems to resent that the customer is going on vacation while she isn't. These hostile feelings cloud her judgement about what to say.

How Did the Communication Strategies Affect the Outcome?

Leslie inadvertently misled Mr. Audette. Her opening explanation made the situation sound very simple, as if verifying which type of Anusol was all the information the pharmacy needed to fill the prescription. Naturally, when Mr. Audette supplied the answer, he thought he was all set, but then Leslie told him that his word wasn't good enough. Leslie tried to make the customer feel guilty by snidely reminding him that he has had the prescription for three days. She attempted to fix the blame on him instead of stepping back to formulate a better explanation of why her hands were tied. By the end of the interaction she seemed to have taken the whole incident personally.

How Could This Have Been Handled Differently?

Obviously, Leslie didn't need to throw in that hostile crack about waiting three days to fill the prescription. If the patient didn't need it, what's the crime in waiting until it's convenient? At least he had the Rx dropped off in advance. Perhaps if Leslie had said something like: "You know, I wish that I could take your word for it and fill your prescription right away. I can see that you're in a hurry; unfortunately, my hands are tied by a pharmacy law that requires me to wait for authorization and clarification. I've tried to reach your doctor a few times; let me try again right now because I don't want to hold you up. . . ." If Leslie proceeds in this manner, at least the patient can bear witness to the efforts she is making on his behalf and the sincerity with which she regrets his inconvenience.

"I'M SORRY, BUT WE ARE OUT OF STOCK ON YOUR MEDS"

Background

It is Friday morning in the Veteran Administration Hospital outpatient pharmacy. It is a high volume pharmacy where the doctors write more prescriptions than the budget can manage and there are chronic problems keeping common drugs in stock. On this particular day a patient has been waiting two hours for a blood pressure medication that turned out to be out of stock.

[Pat's unspoken thoughts are italicized and set off by brackets.]

Pat: "Good morning sir, how may I help you?"

Mr. O'Rourke: "I've been waiting two (expletive) hours for my pills!"

Pat: [*How does one (expletive) for two hours?*] Sir, could you step to the door for a moment?"

Agenda-

Mr. O'Rourke: "Why? I just want my pills so I can get the (expletive) out of here."

Pat: [*We don't have his meds and I am going to have to look him in the eye and tell him. He uses that expletive in so many beautiful ways.*] "I realize it's been a long wait and that is what I want to discuss with you."

Mr. O'Rourke: "Make it quick."

Pat: [*I've got to get the upper hand.*] "I'm sorry but we are out of stock of your meds. When we receive more I will personally mail your Rx to you."

Mr. O'Rourke: "This is my high blood pressure we're talking about!"

Pat: "I realize that and I know you've been waiting a long time but if you go and see your doctor and he dispenses an alternative drug, we can get that right to you."

Mr. O'Rourke: "This place is so (expletive)! If I die it's on your head. You'd better have my medications for me on Monday."

Pat: [*Such a windbag!*] "I'll see to it. Just ask for me and you won't have to wait."

Mr. O'Rourke: "You just better have my drugs!"

Pat: "O.K. Ah . . . have a nice day." [*Good riddance!*]

Case Commentary

What Happened?

Pat's objectives were to inform the patient that his meds were temporarily out of stock and that they could be reordered within a few days. Pat wasn't looking for a fight and certainly did not want to hassle Mr. O'Rourke. Any pharmacist who has worked or interned in a V.A. hospital realizes that the veterans always need more goods and services than the system can provide. Tension runs high at most veteran hospitals.

How Did Unspoken Thoughts and Assumptions
Affect the Interaction?

Pat is obviously shocked by Mr. O'Rourke's gruff manner and use of profanity. In fact, Pat seems a bit intimidated by him and their conversation quickly turns into a power struggle. Pat experiences Mr. O'Rourke's desperation as nothing more than a dramatic act designed to get attention. This belief that Mr. O'Rourke is exaggerating keeps Pat from feeling any compassion for him. Having lost his patience, Pat feels justified in saying anything to get rid of him for the moment.

How Did the Communication Strategies Affect the Outcome?

This was a bad situation that could have been made worse if it had been more public. Pat was wise to pull Mr. O'Rourke aside to deliver the bad news. Pat tried to deliver a minimal amount of empathy, "I realize that it's been a long wait . . . ," but somehow this seemed like too hollow and insincere a gesture to Mr. O'Rourke. Perhaps Mr. O'Rourke sensed that Pat was gratuitously "easing in" to dropping the bomb of bad news. Paradoxically, trying to soften the blow increases the tension. Pat's promise to personally fill Mr. O'Rourke's prescription on Monday raises the question of whether or not he is scheduled to work that day. Trying to defer an unpleasant situation is not an uncommon conflict management style. Pat also should have shown some effort and initiative by offering to call the doctor for an alternative Rx. Telling Mr. O'Rourke to go back upstairs makes it seem like Pat hasn't heard a word Mr. O'Rourke has said about being tired of waiting.

How Could This Have Been Handled Differently?

As a result of Pat's poor communication skills, Mr. O'Rourke left the pharmacy both unhappy and without any medication. His health could be in serious jeopardy. Pat should have started the conversation with the most important fact first. He could have said: "I'm concerned about helping you control your blood pressure and that's why I am not happy to have to tell you that we are out of your particular medication. Before you leave here, I need to make sure that you have enough to take until our new stock comes in, because if not, I need to call upstairs to get your doctor to write an alternative prescription. . . ." Pat also needs to acknowledge Mr. O'Rourke's frustration with waiting around the hospital, perhaps by adding: "I know the last thing you wanted to hear right now is there will be a further delay with your medication. . . ." Speaking directly to the patient's irritation will help manage the situation effectively.

"WHAT? I CAN'T BELIEVE THIS!"

Background

It is Saturday and Mrs. Jack arrives with a prescription from the hospital's ambulatory walk-in clinic. As usual, it was at least a twenty-minute wait because of the backup. The prescription was for a cream which was previously stocked in tubes but is no longer.

[Brian's unspoken thoughts are italicized and set off by brackets.]

Brian: "Good morning, may I help you?"

Mrs. Jack: "I have been waiting for the pediatrician for an hour and a half. I'm sick and tired of this place. The service is horrible. Here's the prescription."

Brian: [*She looks like major trouble.*] "O.K. Does your little guy have any allergies?"

Mrs. Jack: "Enough with the questions! Are you going to fill this or not? If so, how long is the wait?"

Brian: [*She's so pushy!*] "About 15 minutes. Have a seat and we will call you. (Exactly 15 minutes later) . . . Mrs. Jack, here is your Lotrimin cream."

Mrs. Jack: "What? I can't believe this!"

Brian: [*I'm shocked–what's wrong?*] "Excuse me?"

Mrs. Jack: "This isn't the first time I bought this cream and I never got these obscene-looking vials."

Brian: "We used to stock this in tubes." [*She's getting me upset. What else can I say?*]

Mrs. Jack: "Listen young man. I went to nursing school and worked as a nurse. I know this simply is not sanitary!"

Brian: [*She's screaming at me like I'm a piece of garbage.*] "This is the only way we carry this cream."

Mrs. Jack: "I demand to speak to your manager."

Brian: [*She won't listen.*] "I'm sorry, she won't be in this morning."

Mrs. Jack: "Give me my prescription back–I'm going someplace else."

Case Commentary

What Happened?

Mrs. Jack was very shocked by the change in appearance of her prescription. Brian never addressed her alarm, and therefore, she never calmed down. Of course, Mrs. Jack was already worked up and ready to react because of her negative experience in pediatrics and her general state of mind was never addressed. A little empathy may have gone a long way in keeping her from exploding.

How Did Unspoken Thoughts and Assumptions Affect the Interaction?

From the first sight of Mrs. Jack, Brian decided that she was going to be trouble and no doubt he put his defenses up right away. Because Mrs. Jack was so tired, unhappy, and alarmed, she "took it out" on Brian. Brian's unspoken thoughts indicated that he knew this was happening but he never spoke up to defend his right as a human being not to be verbally abused. It is almost as if Brian assumed that Mrs. Jack was so troubled that she couldn't be reasoned with and so he gave up on trying to empathize and reassure her and instead responded minimally. The "be very quiet and reduce the size of the target" strategy rarely works.

How Did the Communication Strategies Affect the Outcome?

Brian allowed himself to be bullied into a corner. He needed to give Mrs. Jack some responsible, appropriate feedback on how she was treating him. Brian needed to assert at least as much control of the conversation as Mrs. Jack. When Mrs. Jack told him basically to shut up (e.g., "Enough with these questions"), Brian needed to respond with empathy but also with a firm explanation about why medical questions are necessary and cannot be avoided. Perhaps Brian could have deflected some of Mrs. Jack's anger through partial agreement. He could have acknowledged that it is annoying when the hospital is understaffed. He also could have conceded that the vials for the cream are not as attractive as the tubes.

How Could This Have Been Handled Differently?

Brian needs to start with some basic empathy to let Mrs. Jack know she is being listened to. When she came storming in full of complaints, a simple "It looks like you have had a hard day" might help. Of course this might elicit a bit more frustration before she calms down. She might respond, "Hard day, let me tell you, there were ten thousand kids screaming their heads off up in Pediatrics! My daughter was fine before I took her up and now she's crying too." Brian needs to keep up the empathy and perhaps respond with, "So, when you take her somewhere to get her feeling better and you both come out feeling worse, you must wonder if it was worth it at all," to which Mrs. Jack might say "Exactly," if she is ready. If not, she'll have to cycle through with a few more complaints. As long as her statements are met with empathy, she will eventually settle down.

Additionally, Brian should defend the pharmacy's reputation when Mrs. Jack accuses him of dispensing unsanitary products. He needs to say, "Although I am sure you didn't intend to communicate this, when you say our products are unsanitary, it makes me feel that you think I would jeopardize your child's health and welfare. I can assure you, we never compromise the delivery of our medications, although I agree the appearance is less than ideal."

Speaking to the unspoken dynamics and acknowledging the truth in tough situations is an essential skill.

"YES, BUT I DIDN'T THINK IT WOULD BE THIS MUCH"

Background

As a benefit to the retired employees, the hospital pharmacy fills their prescriptions. Mrs. Prout is one such retiree with a history of pushing the system by requesting lots of "favors." This time Mrs. Prout wants a special brand of aerosol inhalant that is not kept in inventory. Marie agreed to special-order it for her and warned her it would not be at the lower contract price that the other inhaler was. Mrs. Prout agreed to take a three-month supply and was instructed to come during a weekday since the hospital department of pharmacy can't handle cash or checks and items must be paid for at the cashier's office. Mrs. Prout arrives on an understaffed Saturday afternoon.

[Marie's unspoken thoughts are italicized and set off by brackets.]

Mrs. Prout: "Hi, I'm here for my husband's prescription.

Marie: [*Not on the day you're supposed to come.*] "Hello, Mrs. Prout. Everything is all set."

Mrs. Prout: "This bill is a lot higher than last time."

Marie: [*I can't believe this.*] "Don't you recall our discussion that this brand was no longer on contract and would be higher?"

Mrs. Prout: "Yes, but I didn't think it would be this much!"

Marie: [*Let's try a different tactic, I don't want to have to return these inhalers for credit. Why did I agree to this in the first place?*] "Your husband needs this for his treatments. We special-ordered a three month supply for him as we agreed."

Mrs. Prout: "He has enough for now. Just refill his prescription with the brand you have. I'll be back on Tuesday."

Case Commentary

What Happened?

Marie anticipated having no problems at all in fulfilling the earlier agreement and dispensing the medication as expediently as possible. She assumed that any questions and concerns that Mrs. Prout might have would have come up in their earlier conversation. Why was Marie wrong in assuming there would be no conflict?

How Did Unspoken Thoughts and Assumptions Affect the Interaction?

Because Marie assumed the agreement was explicit, she was caught off guard by Mrs. Prout's objections. It is a very human trait to get very quiet when we are stunned by something and we are trying to figure out how to respond. Marie is already a few steps ahead in wondering if she can return the special order for credit, when the conflict at hand hasn't yet been fully discussed. Marie also obviously assumed that money was not as important to Mrs. Prout as brand loyalty. In the end Marie is kicking herself and is ready to submit her name for "wimp of the year."

How Did the Communication Strategies Affect the Outcome?

Marie must have felt that Mrs. Prout didn't listen to her in their first conversation and that she wasn't listening to her again. But if Marie puts all the blame on Mrs. Prout's poor skills, she is missing out on an opportunity to improve her own. Looking back on Marie's statements, it is easy to infer that she has a problem with being specific and direct. When she says, "Don't you recall our discussion that the brand was no longer on contract and would be higher?" Marie doesn't say that she told Mrs. Prout exactly how much more the cost would be. The word "higher" is too abstract in this case and Mrs. Prout may have thought that higher meant a few cents more. Did Marie fail to be specific with her because she was uncomfortable talking about money with this retiree? Was she hoping Mrs. Prout would say, "Forget it, I guess I can take another brand to save money''? When she didn't say this, Marie went ahead with the extra effort of the special order hoping everything would turn out okay.

How Could This Have Been Handled Differently?

Obviously in the first conversation Marie needed to state the exact price difference per inhaler refill. Given that this didn't happen, she needed to take ownership for her lack of specificity. She needed to say something like, "Mrs. Prout, I can tell from your shock about the price that I wasn't clear enough about the cost difference the last time we talked and I'm sorry for that. . . . Still, this presents a bit of a problem. Although it may be possible to return this special order for credit, if it doesn't present too much of a financial hardship, I am wondering if we can come to some agreement about your purchase of the order we placed for you and then discuss exactly what we should do in the future." By telling Mrs. Prout more of what is going through her mind, Marie increases the chances that they can work effectively together toward a compromise.

Chapter 6

Counseling Patients in the Hospital

"DOES EACH OF YOUR DOCTORS KNOW WHAT THE OTHER IS GIVING YOU?"

Background

Lynn is on duty in the outpatient pharmacy on Saturday and she recognizes Ms. Bennet because she dispensed Tylox to her just the day before. Ms. Bennet presents a script for Percodan.

[Lynn's unspoken thoughts are italicized and set off by brackets.]

Lynn: [*Red alert–conflict.*] "I'm sorry Ms. Bennet. Since I filled your Tylox prescription yesterday I cannot fill this prescription for you today."

Ms. Bennet: "Why not?"

Lynn: "Both are pain relievers and yesterday you got enough for five days."

Ms. Bennet: "So?"

Lynn: "These prescriptions are from different doctors. Does each know what the other is writing for?"

Ms. Bennet: "Yes. They work at this same hospital, don't they?"

Lynn: [*Oops, I think I led her into that. Is this lady a doctor hopper?*] "I cannot fill this for you. Get in touch with your doctor when the Tylox is gone."

Ms. Bennet: "You cannot refuse me. You are only a pharmacist."

Lynn: [*She looks desperate.*] "Both drugs work in the same way in your body. Without being able to get in touch with both doctors I am afraid to give you more of the same thing."

Ms. Bennet: "But I really need it." (crying)

Case Commentary

What Happened?

Lynn tried to tell Ms. Bennet why she could not have the medication that she wanted. The pharmacist's attempt wasn't awful but it wasn't a full, complete, and motivating explanation either. Lynn never determined whether Ms. Bennet is a chronic drug abuser or a desperate person in a lot of pain.

*How Did Unspoken Thoughts and Assumptions
Affect the Interaction?*

Lynn knew there was a potential conflict from the very beginning. She was wondering if Ms. Bennet was deliberately switching from doctor to doctor, and yet she never was able to ask about it in such a way as to get a comprehensive answer. Ms. Bennet sounded almost insulting to Lynn, but because the pharmacist kept in mind the fact that she was desperate, Lynn was able to avoid getting hooked by her remarks. This interaction was rather drawn out and it seems that Lynn thought that Ms. Bennet would see the pharmacist's view and drop the matter in short order.

How Did the Communication Strategies Affect the Outcome?

Lynn should have been tipped off to her own ineffectiveness by Ms. Bennet's sequence of cryptic questions. The inquiries of "So?" and "Why not?" indicate that Lynn has not given an adequate explanation of why she has to say no. This is not the time to launch into long explanations of the pharmacy laws and policies that prohibit dispensing. Rather, Lynn needs to focus on her concern for

Ms. Bennet's health and drug therapy. She needs to be explicit about what the effect would be if Ms. Bennet took both prescriptions simultaneously. A more active response than "Get in touch with your doctor when this is gone" was called for.

How Could This Have Been Handled Differently?

Lynn needed to be more direct from the very beginning by saying something like "I'm very concerned about how you're feeling, Ms. Bennet, because I see that you're bringing in a second prescription from a different doctor that virtually duplicates the effect of the medicine you picked up yesterday." . . . "I could be wrong, but I'm wondering if you're in so much pain that you thought that taking two types of pain reliever would make you feel better in half the time or take away more of the pain." . . . "The reason I can't fill this for you is because if you took both types of drugs together it would be too much for your body." . . . "I hate to see you in so much pain so perhaps you'll allow me to call both doctors and we can decide what drug therapy will bring you the maximum relief. . . ." Without this additional counseling, Ms. Bennet may not realize that she could be putting herself at risk.

"I CAN SEE THIS IS REALLY UPSETTING TO YOU"

Background

Walt is on duty on a Saturday at an H.M.O. pharmacy when a young woman approaches with an empty package of birth control pills.

[Walt's unspoken thoughts are italicized and set off by brackets.]

Ms. Chirtie: "I need more of these."

Walt: [*She looks unhappy and teary eyed.*] "Just let me check the computer to see if you have a refill coming. (Computer indicates that woman's H.M.O. is rejecting claims.) I'm afraid there is a problem with your insurance; you will have to pay with cash for your refill."

Ms. Chirtie: "I've had this problem before, but I thought it was worked out."

Walt: [*What can I do with a crying woman?*] "I can see this is really upsetting to you. I am sorry that you are stuck in the middle of an administrative problem."

Ms. Chirtie: (starting to cry more) "I don't want to go off my pills but I don't have twenty dollars."

Walt: [*I feel helpless.*] "I wish I could help."

Ms. Chirtie: "I don't understand why this is happening."

Case Commentary

What Happened?

This was a very difficult situation to handle. Walt avoided making it into a worse one by refraining from the usual, "Well, didn't you pay your bills?" type of response. Obviously, if the woman can't pay for her pills, the pharmacy can't give them to her for free. In this type of situation anything that Walt said was bound to provoke an emotional reaction. If Walt hadn't been so empathic, it is very likely that he also would have gotten yelled at for hassling and insulting the patient.

How Did the Unspoken Thoughts and Assumptions
Affect the Interaction?

Walt felt really helpless when Ms. Chirtie started to cry. What would have happened if he felt "manipulated" instead? He probably would have grown angry with her and what good would that have done? She no doubt would sense his displeasure with her and begin to get defensive. Instead, Walt kept the focus on himself, wondering to no avail what he could do to help. If he further thought, "Who would actually cry over the small amount required to get a birth control refill?" he would take himself further away from where he needs to be to feel empathy for her. Maybe she uses the birth control to regulate her menstrual cycle. Maybe she is worried about being able to afford other needed health care services. If Walt assumes she is in deep self-pity over the fate of her sex life, he will have a difficult time interacting effectively with her.

How Did the Communication Strategies Affect the Outcome?

Although Walt was fairly empathic, he could have gone a bit further at times. He was somewhat abrupt and unsympathetic when he informed her of her "cash only" option. When Ms. Chirtie said that she has had this problem before but thought it had been worked out, Walt failed to inquire about her understanding of the situation. Perhaps she had recently paid a premium and the computer does not reflect it yet. Offering to pick up the phone to call the central financial office would at least show some effort on Walt's part. Still, it was good that Walt validated how "stuck" Ms. Chirtie felt not knowing how to resolve the problem.

How Could This Have Been Handled Differently?

It would probably have helped if Walt had said something like, "I'm puzzled as to why I can't get your claim through on your insurance, but perhaps you know something about this?" ... "This isn't going to make you happy and perhaps it is unfair if this is a foul-up on the part of the company, but I am afraid I have to ask you to pay cash for your prescription." ... "Would you like me to call the central office to find out why this is happening?" ... "I am really frustrated myself because I don't know how to make this better for you right now. ...." By continuing to take her concerns seriously and by being willing to make extra efforts, Walt could show his dedication to quality patient care.

"THIS COSTS TOO MUCH FOR SOMEONE ON A FIXED INCOME"

Background

Arnie is on duty at the outpatient pharmacy in the city hospital. An elderly woman arrives from the ambulatory clinic.

[Arnie's unspoken thoughts are italicized and set off by brackets.]

Arnie: "Hi, can I help you?"

Mrs. Ray: "My doctor called you to get my refills ready. I'm Mrs. Ray."

Arnie: [*This should be no problem.*] "I have Propranocol and Diazide here for you."

Mrs. Ray: "Yes, that's it."

Arnie: "Have you taken these before?"

Mrs. Ray: "Oh, yes."

Arnie: [*So she's used to this price.*] "Okay. That will be $45.00."

Mrs. Ray: "This costs too much for someone on a fixed income."

Arnie: [*My grandmother has been having a hard time too.*] "Yes, it's awful. I don't know how people on fixed incomes keep up."

Mrs. Ray: "It's very tough. I don't know how much longer I'll be able to keep paying!"

Arnie: [*I wonder what kind of sacrifices she has to make to come up with this money?*] "It is very scary."

Mrs. Ray: "It just seems like nobody understands how hard it is."

Case Commentary

What Happened?

Arnie handled this situation fairly well simply by "staying in the moment" with Mrs. Ray. He kept the focus on Mrs. Ray instead of being distracted by his own concerns, e.g., "I know what you mean, my car insurance has skyrocketed." Arnie did not get defensive and take the complaint personally as many pharmacists do in this situation.

How Did Unspoken Thoughts and Assumptions Affect the Interaction?

Although Arnie validated Mrs. Ray's shock over the price of the medication, he also should have taken the time to verify whether or not Mrs. Ray understood how to take these very expensive drugs. His simple "Have you taken this before?" is a closed-ended question that calls for a minimal response. An open ended question would provide information as to whether or not Mrs. Ray was taking her medicine correctly. The elderly often under-dose in an attempt to save money, and Arnie should realize that, because of what Mrs. Ray is saying, she is "at risk" unless he verifies how she is taking this medication.

How Did the Communication Strategies Affect the Outcome?

In a societal atmosphere that rejects aging, pharmacists must be very sensitive to the feelings of the elderly who frequent pharmacies. The elderly often have physical problems, mental health problems, financial problems, and issues with social isolation. Arnie seems to intuitively recognize Mrs. Ray's multiple burdens and at the very least manages not to add to them. Whereas many pharmacists become visibly upset with elderly customers who question prices, Arnie refuses to hear Mrs. Ray's concerns as a "complaint," and instead actively tries to identify with her concerns. The reality of the elderly on fixed incomes is very harsh. They often have to decide whether it is better to have money for food or medication. Arnie continues to recognize these stresses and therefore avoids the all too common response: "I don't set the prices ma'am; you're welcome to try a retail store."

How Could This Have Been Handled Differently?

There are a few practical steps that Arnie may have overlooked. For example, is the hospital's profit margin sufficient that he can offer a ten percent discount as many retail shops do? The extra four dollars in Mrs. Ray's pocket may mean a meal she wouldn't have to miss and it shows real effort and concern on Arnie's part. Similarly, are all of Mrs. Ray's drugs being offered in generics? Arnie can offer to call upstairs to get authorization to switch products if it will save some money. Also, many pharmaceutical company have programs for the indigent. More importantly, Arnie should not allow Mrs. Ray to leave before verifying that she will take her medicines properly. As suggested by the Indian Health Care Patient Consultation Program (see Chapter One), Arnie should either rephrase his closed-ended question or follow up with an open-ended question: "Just to make sure I haven't missed anything, could you tell me how you are going to take your medication?" By providing practical help, double-checking her compliance, and showing empathy for her concerns, Arnie would be doing all that he could to serve Mrs. Ray effectively.

"I HAVE TO GO GET ANOTHER CHEMO TREATMENT"

Background

A major teaching hospital maintains an outpatient chemotherapy clinic which is basically a room with six long chairs with a suspended TV to help pass the time. The outpatient pharmacy is next to the chemo room and the pharmacists come to know the patients quite well as they come by to pick up narcotics, anti-emetics, vials, and needles. On this particular day, Carrie is alone on duty in the pharmacy.

[Carrie's unspoken thoughts are italicized and set off by brackets.]

Mr. Clancy: "I have to go get another chemo treatment in a few minutes. I don't understand why I have to come back here so much. You'd think that all that other medicine I take would help."

Carrie: [*Poor guy looks exhausted.*] "It must be very hard on you to have to come in so often. It takes a lot of time out of your daily activities."

Mr. Clancy: "Not only that, I feel so sick afterward."

Carrie: "You seem discouraged; is there anything I can do?"

Mr. Clancy: "I've heard marijuana helps with the pain. But my doctor says it would be illegal. He doesn't understand how sick I get."

Carrie: [*I don't want to get into a debate over legalities.*] "So you feel like he doesn't understand how desperate you feel?"

Mr. Clancy: "He's a good doctor, but he doesn't feel the pain I do."

Carrie: [*I wish he'd try explaining things to his doctor again.*] "It seems like you think he doesn't understand how out of control this pain has gotten."

Mr. Clancy: "I guess he is trying his best, but I'd like him to understand why I would do anything to feel better."

Case Commentary

What Happened?

Fighting cancer can sometimes destroy all the hope and faith that people have in their own futures. Many chemotherapy patients quit their treatment because the side effects become unbearable. Carrie allowed Mr. Clancy to express his feelings of pain and discouragement without giving him the false hope that he will be cured soon or that marijuana will be the answer to all his problems.

How Did Unspoken Thoughts and Assumptions Affect the Interaction?

Carrie clearly feels bad for Mr. Clancy. She is listening with her eyes as well as her ears as she notices how depleted he looks. Although she knows she cannot take away all of his problems, she at least resolves consciously not to add to his burdens. She realizes that it would be futile to get into a debate about whether or not T.H.C. should be more available to cancer patients. In fact, getting into this type of "intellectual" discussion brings both parties away from the feelings that need to be felt in the moment. If Carrie had said: "Those darn bureaucrats at the F.D.A. just don't understand, do they?" it would have taken Mr. Clancy away from one of the sources of his pain, which was his basic feeling of not being sympathized with by his doctor. Most likely other members of his health care team in addition to his doctor are not allowing him to fully vent his feelings of desperation.

How Did the Communication Strategies Affect the Outcome?

Carrie listened to Mr. Clancy and reflected back to him the fact that she understands. This reflection of feeling enables him to vent more of his pain, whereas if she had prematurely tried to placate, give advice, judge, or cross-examine him, he would not have felt free to continue to talk. This process is similar to the cleansing of a physical wound. We always wash off the scrape before putting the bandage on top, and similarly, Mr. Clancy needs to cleanse himself by talking about his anxieties before he will be able to continue to comply with his treatment plan. Carrie stayed right with Mr. Clancy in his moment of pain. She didn't try to distract him or change the subject as most people tend to do. She showed a lot of sensitivity and perhaps this is a reflection on her own evolution of thinking about human suffering and life-threatening illness.

How Could This Have Been Handled Differently?

As previously mentioned, Carrie did a good job being present with Mr. Clancy, but there are a few more actions she can take. She can offer to talk with his doctor about his nausea medication. Carrie can ask Mr. Clancy if he would like her suggestions and opinions on what to say to his doctor. Carrie can offer to brainstorm with Mr. Clancy. For instance, would changes in diet or going for therapeutic massage help him better manage the pain? It is important, however, that Carrie resist jumping right into the problem-solving, advice-giving role without first explicitly discussing with Mr. Clancy if he wants to focus on the options. It could be that all Mr. Clancy needs today is for someone to simply understand his pain.

"WHERE ARE MY COLOSTOMY BAGS?"

Background

Mr. Victor has been coming into the hospital outpatient pharmacy every day for the past week to try to obtain his colostomy bags. There has been a manufacturer's delay and the pharmacist has provided similar bags to tie him over for the next week.

[Dale's unspoken thoughts are italicized and set off by brackets.]

Mr. Victor: "Where are my colostomy bags?"

Dale: [*I can't believe he's back!*] "I'm sorry, Mr. Vale, but like I told you yesterday, they aren't in yet."

Mr. Victor: "I have arthritis and I can't keep coming in like this."

Dale: "You don't have to; I'll call you at home the moment they arrive." [*Please stop coming in.*]

Mr. Victor: "I'm down to my last bag; this isn't a pleasant experience."

Dale: [*What's the problem?*] "I get the sense that you don't want to try some of the substitute bags I gave you."

Mr. Victor: "This is an emergency case. You don't know what I'm going through."

Dale: [*Why won't he just try?*] "I guess it's uncomfortable for you to use the others because they are not an exact fit."

Mr. Victor: "I'm really desperate!"

Dale: "I wish I could be more helpful."

Case Commentary

What Happened?

Dale does not seem very sympathetic to Mr. Victor's problem. It seems that by promising Mr. Victor that he will get the bags as soon as humanly possible, Dale thinks he has done all he can for the patient. When pharmacists get frustrated over their own inability to be helpful, their communication with the patient often becomes ineffective.

How Did Unspoken Thoughts and Assumptions Affect the Interaction?

Dale seems somewhat frustrated with Mr. Victor's persistence. He wonders why Mr. Victor will not do as he is told and stay at home until he is called, like a "good patient." This focus on "Why is he causing problems?" makes it unlikely that Dale can empathize effectively with his patient. Dale wonders "Why wouldn't he just try the other bags?" and yet he never asks this aloud. There very well could be a good reason why he does not try them or perhaps he has tried them and he was uncomfortable. With such minimal communication, how can Dale truly understand Mr. Victor's current condition?

How Did the Communication Strategies Affect the Outcome?

This situation could definitely have been much worse. Dale resisted overtly judging his patient, although his covert assumptions kept him from being more effective. Dale did not help decrease Mr. Victor's stress level, but he did not really increase it either. Dale attempts to reflect the message behind Mr. Victor's words, but stops short of acknowledging the depth of feeling. By the time Dale expresses his frustration at not being able to help, it is definitely "too little, too late."

How Could This Have Been Handled Differently?

Phrases such as "Like I told you . . ." are punishing and should be avoided. Dale should rephrase himself using ownership language such as "Perhaps I didn't communicate clearly enough about when I expect the colostomy bags to arrive . . ." and more directly, "Yes, I also worry about you aggravating your arthritis if you keep making extra trips; what is it that I can say or do to reassure you that I will call you the second the bags come in?" By asking this open-ended question, Dale puts the burden of explanation on Mr. Victor and thus he will be able to verify whether or not his message is being received. If his message is not getting across, the answers to these types of open-ended questions will enable Dale to assess why he and Mr. Victor are not communicating effectively.

Chapter 7

Conflict with Co-Workers in the Hospital

"I'M NOT HERE TO PLACE EVERY MED IN YOUR HAND FOR YOU"

Background

Thomas is working the 3 to 11 p.m. shift at a suburban hospital. As usual, there is too much work to do and only a skeleton crew. At 5:30 the pharmacy receives a phone call from one of the floors.

[Thomas' unspoken thoughts are italicized and set off by brackets.]

Thomas: "Pharmacy, Thomas speaking. Can I help you?"

Nurse: "I hope so. This is Dina on 4 South. I need a bag of Mr. Black's Ceftriaxone that is due at 6:00 p.m. Will you be bringing it up on the next set of rounds?"

Thomas: [*I did that order myself.*] "I brought that up on the 4:30 rounds. I put it in his box myself, Room 412. Could you check again?" [*They lost it.*]

Nurse: "I already looked and I don't have time to fix your mistakes. Send up another so that the patient does not have to suffer for your mistakes."

Thomas: [*I'd like to reach over the phone line and choke her.*] "That is very expensive medicine. Please check again; I'm positive it's there."

Nurse: "I don't have time. Just bring it up. Bye."
(Hangs up.)

(Thomas prepares the I.V. and arrives on the floor and sees the other I.V. right where he said it would be.)

Thomas: (Loudly) "Dina? Dina? Is there a Dina on this floor?" [*Let's see her get out of this one.*]

Nurse: "I'm right here. Do you have my medicine?"

Thomas: [*That's it!*] "I sure do, you incompetent witch! If you hadn't been so arrogant on the phone and taken 15 seconds to look like I asked you to you would have had it 30 minutes ago. It was right where I said, so what's your excuse?"

Nurse: "We were so busy and I didn't think it had come up yet."

Thomas: "We're busy downstairs, too. I'm not here to place every med in your hands for you. That's what these boxes are for–so you don't have to go searching. But you're too stupid to even do that right. The worst thing is that Mr. Black suffers because he has to pay for your incompetence. We have to charge for the second dose." [*I've got her now. I wish it had come out of her salary.*]

Nurse: "Hey, it's not my fault."

Thomas: (cutting her off) "So I suppose it's mine? The next time you need something from the pharmacy, be prepared to wait a long time for it." [*Maybe I've gone a bit too far but she deserves it.*]

Case Commentary

What Happened?

No doubt Thomas had a few relatively simple objectives early on in this confrontation. He wanted the nurse to look again to save him the trip and he wanted to avoid double-billing an expensive medication. Instead, Thomas has probably triggered off a full-scale war by embarrassing the nurse, who will in turn recruit all of the other nurses to make Thomas's life very difficult. The nurse baited Thomas with her "We're busy and more important than you" attitude and he took it, hook, line, and sinker.

*How Did Unspoken Thoughts and Assumptions
Affect the Interaction?*

If Thomas automatically assumed that the nurses lost the medication, obviously some sort of similar negative pattern between the unit nurses and the pharmacy staff has been established. It is very common for hospital pharmacists to believe that the nurses constantly lose and switch medications and tempers run high around this chronic problem. Toward the end of the confrontation, even Thomas thinks he has gone too far, but he never acknowledges this out loud. He is intent on punishing the nurse in as public a way as possible.

How Did the Communication Strategies Affect the Outcome?

Thomas sends the nurse mixed messages. On the one hand, he tries to make her feel guilty about the cost of the medication and he chides her for making the patient suffer. On the other hand, he tells her that when she needs something important from the pharmacy she is going to have to wait a long time for it. Now who really suffers if he plays a petty game like that? Instead of simply being angry and exploding, he needed to tell the nurse exactly *why* he was angry. After all, no one likes to be "jerked around" and belittled in status and importance. Clearly, the nurse sent Thomas this exact message. He pushes the nurse into a corner and she is left with "It's not my fault," when clearly they both need to sit down and talk rationally about why "missing" meds is such an ongoing problem.

How Could This Have Been Handled Differently?

Thomas needed to talk to Dina alone and in a quiet tone of voice. Creating a comfortable setting can eliminate a lot of the need for face-saving behavior. Thomas needed to say: "When you demand a new medication delivery without checking on where your current meds are, I feel like you send me the message that your time is more important than mine. . . . This incident seems to be part of an ongoing problem between our departments; I know we in pharmacy are concerned about lost or switched medications. Is there something about the box delivery system that is unclear or doesn't work for you? I know that you are busy up here, so it's likely that you wouldn't notice a pharmacist making deliveries. Since this is the case, can we make an agreement that you will look where the pharmacy staff suggests before duplicating a stat medication?" By negotiating with the nurse and allowing her to respond to each question or statement, Thomas avoids being a doormat and gains a better understanding of the problem, ensuring that the patient care delivery system won't be impaired by interpersonal retaliation strategies, a key issue in hospital practice.

"DIDN'T I MENTION SOMETHING ABOUT A STAT MED I WAS COMING FOR?"

Background

It is a busy morning in the hospital pharmacy and everyone but the order-entry pharmacist and Rick are on break. Rick had taken a call from a doctor who made it clear he was short on time and wanted his med ready when he came for it.

(Dr. Kildare appears at the window and lets himself into the pharmacy.)

[Rick's unspoken thoughts are italicized and set off by brackets.]

Dr. Kildare: "Are you the one I called the Vancomycin order to?"

Rick: "Yes."

Dr. Kildare: "Is it ready?"

Rick: [*He's gonna let me have it.*] "Not exactly sir, you see . . ." (cut off abruptly)

Dr. Kildare: "When did I call this order down?"

Rick: [*What a jerk!*] "15 minutes ago?"

Dr. Kildare: (sarcastically) "Didn't I mention *something* about a stat med I was coming for?"

Rick: [*I hate it when people talk to me this way.*] "Yes, but it's been busy and I'm . . ."

Dr. Kildare: (coughs loudly and looks at watch)

Rick: (goes to stockroom and returns with medication)

Dr. Kildare: "Make sure it's right; I don't have time for you to be fishing around back there."

Rick: "Sorry about this. I hope that next time . . ." [*I'm not really sorry now.*]

Dr. Kildare: "There won't be a next time."

Rick: "Well, have a good one." (sarcastically) [*I'm really angry, like I mean it.*]

Dr. Kildare: (no reply, leaves pharmacy)

Case Commentary

What Happened?

Rick took a lot of unnecessary verbal abuse from Dr. Kildare. Although there is no excuse for the doctor's bullying, we can't do anything about his behavior; we can only focus on the pharmacist's response. In this case, Rick was far too passive regarding Dr. Kildare's punishing statements. Rick never even seized an opportunity to explain why the order wasn't ready.

How Did Unspoken Thoughts and Assumptions Affect the Interaction?

Rick was afraid from the moment that the doctor arrived at the pharmacy. He thought that he was about to get yelled at and indeed that is what happened. People have a way of picking up on and sensing unspoken thoughts and Rick was obviously giving off an "I'm a doormat, walk all over me" message. Rick thought to himself, "I hate it when people talk to me this way!" and yet he couldn't find an effective way to say this out loud. Often aggressive people don't even realize how abusive they are being unless they get feedback on their behavior. It is better to let the bully know that he/she is displaying unacceptable behavior than to simply cower through the experience and try to retaliate later (e.g., perhaps through "creative means" like getting all of your co-workers to "stonewall" the bully).

How Did the Communication Strategies Affect the Outcome?

Rick needed to start with a "preemptive" communication strategy (not the same as a "preemptive strike" of course; we are trying to get away from wars, not start them). Rick should have been the first person to mention that the drug was not ready yet and acknowledge that the delay presents an inconvenience to the doctor. Rick allowed the doctor to entrap him with a series of leading questions (e.g., "When did I call the order down?"). Instead of asserting himself as a person who is not superhuman but is trying hard, Rick stumbles over his words in a rather pathetic attempt at self-defense. By the end of the exchange, all Rick can manage is a note of sarcasm instead of saying something that might help him regain a sense of dignity.

How Could This Have Been Handled Differently?

Rick needed to stop the aggressiveness directed at him. First of all, when he knew the doctor was likely to be unhappy with him he needed to be the one to say it first. "Oh, Dr. Kildare, I know this isn't going to make you happy but I need to explain why the preparation of your medication was delayed. . . ." And if Dr. Kildare persisted in making a fuss Rick needed to say: "I can see that you're angry, but when you criticize me harshly without fully understanding my situation, I find it hard to continue working effectively with you. . . ." If things still end with a pseudo-threat Rick could say: "When you say "There won't be a next time" it makes me feel bad about my sincere attempt to be of service; can we talk about what just happened here?" By explaining other communication options, Rick can prevent himself from being blamed and possibly establish a better relationship with the doctor.

"WOULD YOU MIND MAKING IVs?"

Background

Kate is in charge of running the IV Room although it is only her second day in the position. Karen and Elaine are her staff for the day and Karen has many years of experience working in the sterile products area.

[Kate's unspoken thoughts are italicized and set off by brackets.]

Kate: "Karen, would you mind making IVs inside? Elaine is going to check off IVs for the morning delivery when she comes in."

Karen: "I can do the checking off. I've done it all before."

Kate: [*She doesn't have as much experience as Elaine and this isn't the day for practice.*] "I was told to have Elaine do it 'cause she usually does it."

Karen: "I know how, too, and I don't have a full crew tomorrow so I'll need to practice doing it for then."

Kate: "O.K. I'll have Elaine do IVs instead."

Karen: "Where's the big cart for the IV bins?"

Kate: "It's out there with stuff on it. It would be easier to use the smaller carts."

Karen: "We always use the big cart in the morning."

Kate: "But that's for the weekdays when one person delivers all the I.V.s to the satellites. On the weekends technicians from the satellites come down for their own IVs so it won't matter if you use the smaller cart." [*I can't believe we are arguing over such a trivial thing!*]

Karen: "Elaine? Don't we always use the big cart in the morning?"

Elaine: "Yeah, we do."

Kate: "I just thought it would be less hassle and save you time if you don't have to remove all that stuff from the big cart first." [*In other words, I don't want to get behind schedule.*]

Karen: "It won't take long . . . you haven't finished the fat emulsions yet?"

Kate: "No. Why don't you check off all the IVs first and then the fat emulsions. That way you won't have to go back and forth checking them off one at a time. That's what I was taught to do."

Karen: "I was told that takes up too much time."

Kate: "O.K., if that's how you want to do it." (After three hours Karen finishes the normally two-hour job.)

Karen: "God! This was such a pain!"

Kate: [*Why is she complaining? She's the one who insisted!*] "Sorry I asked you to do the delivery. I guess today wasn't the best day to practice since we don't have a really strong crew, but you insisted."

Karen: "Fine, someone else can work out here with you. I'm a whiz in the IV Room."

Kate: [*She always seems so sure of herself.*] "Yes, you are good, that's why I suggested Elaine do this delivery while you worked here."

Karen: (slams down tray, storms inside IV Room saying loudly . . .) "Someone go out there and label with Kate; I'm not working out there."

Case Commentary

What Happened?

Kate, as a new manager, had the objective of sticking to the department's tight schedule and not making any enemies as she settled into her supervisory position. The situation between Kate and Karen degenerated into a very negative interaction with a lot of resentment seething just below the surface. Kate and Karen have started their new working relationship off on the wrong foot.

How Did Unspoken Thoughts and Assumptions Affect the Interaction?

Kate had a lot of fears in her mind that she didn't share with Karen. She was very worried that she would look bad if the department ran behind scheduling on her second day on the job. What was it that kept her from saying this to Karen? Wouldn't she have solicited sympathy and cooperation if she was honest about what she was thinking? Instead, Kate tries to choose her words so as to maneuver Karen into doing things her way. Karen responds in kind and they continue to "counter-argue" with each other about ways of doing the job.

The situation has become ridiculous in Kate's mind and even she can't believe that they are arguing over which cart to use. What was it that prevented her from saying, "I notice that we are arguing back and forth about procedures, which is slowing us both down even more; my biggest fear is that we will be behind all day. How can we both make sure that doesn't happen?"

How Did the Communication Strategies Affect the Outcome?

There were many things that Karen said that Kate avoided confronting effectively. For example, when Karen said she needed "practice" checking off IVs, Kate did not say what the consequences might be of taking time to practice. On the other hand, when Karen complained about what a pain the job was, Kate confronted her ineffectively by in essence saying "You asked for it." When Karen responds in kind, Kate basically says, "I told you so!" Kate communicates "Don't blame me, you are the problem."

Both women seem to be appealing to the great "they" authority in the sky to bolster their case and to distance themselves from taking responsibility for their thoughts and feelings. Notice the frequency of statements like: "I was told . . . ," "We always use . . . ," "That's what I was taught. . . ." Karen and Kate are going back and forth with each other on what "sounds" like rational reasonable disagreements about procedure, but in actuality they are simply striking out and striking back at each other. For example, after Kate pesters Karen about which cart to use, Karen hits back with the hostile, "Oh, you haven't finished the fat emulsions yet?" In other words, "You're one to talk . . . so get off my back."

How Could This Have Been Handled Differently?

Why not break the negative pattern with a statement like, "It really seems like we are on each other's cases right now. I know I certainly have contributed, but can we start over and plan together how the work can be delegated most effectively?" New managers often feel awkward and are afraid that they will either be perceived as too authoritarian or too laissez faire. What is it that keeps new supervisors from sharing these fears? Wouldn't it be liberating for Kate to be able to say to her co-workers, "While at the same time keeping my eye on the bottom line (time and money concerns), I need your feedback on how to run the department effectively without being too bossy or too much of a pushover."

Participatory management will go further than trying to "control" the staff's behavior. Kate tried to control Karen's behavior through hostile debate and passive aggression and unless they both learn to step back from the situation, they can look forward to more of the same in the future.

"SINCE YOU OBVIOUSLY KNOW SO LITTLE, YOU'D BETTER KEEP YOUR MOUTH SHUT"

Background

The setting is a small satellite pharmacy with six people working in a space designed for two but with a workload for ten. It's hot, the air conditioning is failing, and regular employees are on vacation. Tension is high. Larry is a fairly new pharmacy technician.

[Scott's unspoken thoughts are italicized and set off by brackets.]

Scott: [*I'm going to embarrass this overly authoritative twit like never before.*] "Could you repeat what you just said?"

Larry: "What do you mean?"

Scott: "What I heard you say on the phone about sustained releases?"

Larry: "You know, about Enteric-coated . . ."

Scott: [*I know and you don't.*] "What were you saying about it?"

Larry: "I was saying how you can crush it and it alters the D.O.A."

Scott: "What the hell are you talking about?"

Larry: "If you crush the tablet it will all be in his stomach at once, speeding up absorption."

Scott: "So . . . ?"

Larry: "Don't you get it?"

Scott: [*Let me help him dig his grave.*] "What exactly does Enteric-coated mean?"

Larry: "It has to do with the drug's release."

Scott: "Exactly what about the release of the drug?"

Larry: "How long it takes?"

Scott: [*I'm about to nail him.*] "Due to where it's released or due to some sort of sustained release mechanism?"

Larry: "I'm not exactly sure but . . ."

Scott: "Do you mean you gave out information based on words you were unfamiliar with?"

Larry: "Well, I . . ."

Scott: "Not to mention that as a technician you have no right to give out information to the staff."

Larry: "Well, I thought it had to do with . . ."

Scott: "O.K., does Enteric-coated have to do with sustained action or where the drug is released; pick one!"

Larry: "I guess I think . . . sustained action?"

Scott: [*I've got this know-it-all right where I want him.*] "Wrong!!!

You ignorant fool. You could kill patients and damage the reputation of the pharmacy by giving out false information. Enteric-coated has to do with release location." (Gives full explanation of why)

Larry: "Well, that kinda has to do with release rate."

Scott: [*I'm past my own limits.*] "You idiot! How many times do I have to tell you?"

Larry: "Well, I guess you're right."

Scott: "Of course I'm right and you are never to use a word you don't know in my presence again. Since you obviously know so little, you'd best keep your mouth shut on drug information."

Case Commentary

What Happened?

This case is obviously a situation where too much tension built up over too long a period of time, leading to an inevitable explosion. It is also an extreme version of what the author calls the "Health Care Professional 'Gotcha' Game." All health care professionals, whether nurses, doctors, pharmacists, and so on, have an overlapping body of knowledge. It is common, especially within the hospital system, to hear professionals fighting over issues of who "knows best" about the appropriate treatment or drug for a patient. With all the one-upmanship that goes on, it's a wonder that patients get any care at all! Needless to say, this kind of overly competitive atmosphere leaves everyone feeling brittle. Scott is the very portrait of a burnt-out pharmacist.

How Did Unspoken Thoughts and Assumptions
Affect the Interaction?

Scott has an overly negative view of Larry and this justifies his poor treatment. Larry is a know-it-all in Scott's eyes and apparently there is nothing Scott hates more. It is clear to see that Scott's motivations are not for the good of the patient but rather for his own vindication. All of Scott's unspoken thoughts revolve around the entrapment and maximum embarrassment of Larry. No matter how often we believe that we know somebody *deserves* to be belittled, there are always alternative methods that teach instead of taunt. As it stands now, Larry is likely to go on behaving as he has, while simply taking care to avoid letting Scott eavesdrop on him. He now learns how to hide his ignorance rather than ask for help in learning.

How Did the Communication Strategies Affect the Outcome?

Scott did nothing but ask Larry a series of closed, leading questions designed to help Larry hang himself. In terms of maximum cruelty and building long-term ill will, his strategies were very effective. After Larry helped drive the last nail into his own professional coffin, Scott finished off the job with some good, old-fashioned name-calling. Of course, the exchange was loud enough for all the other staff to hear, which made it an even more important victory for Scott. Scott did not allow Larry even the minimal amount of "face-saving" that most give as a "professional" courtesy.

How Could This Have Been Handled Differently?

First of all, Scott must believe that in the long run, collaboration goes further than competition. If it is part of a pattern for Larry to overstep the bounds of his knowledge, then it is not wrong for his senior pharmacist to reprimand him. The issue is *how* the feedback can be given effectively so that Scott can trust Larry enough to work with him. Scott must start by being more specific. Instead of communicating that Larry *always* gives out bad drug information, Scott needs to detail why Larry has created a crisis of faith in Scott's mind. He needs to say something like: "The other day I heard you fail to ask about a patient's use of aspirin-based OTCs with his prescription Motrin, and yesterday I heard you say that it's okay to mix Diazaide and Lasix, and now today it seems you're confused about what Enteric-coating means. Now it's true that I might simply be focusing on your weaknesses instead of your strengths, but frankly this pattern of basic mistakes has me very concerned. . . . I appreciate your wanting to be helpful to patients and staff but I need you to double-check with me before giving out drug information." Scott would thus resist sending Larry the message that he is "uneducable" and so there would be a better chance that they could continue to work together.

"I'M NOT GOING TO LOSE MY LICENSE OVER THIS"

Background

Anja is on duty in the main hospital pharmacy when a nurse calls down an order for Rocephin–650mg. Anja tells the nurse it will take a few minutes and then she will bring it up.

[Anja's unspoken thoughts are italicized and set off by brackets.]

Anja: "Hi. Here you go." (Hands nurse the syringe)

Nurse: "What's this?"

Anja: [*What do you mean, "What's this?"*] "It's the Rocephin."

Nurse: "You're not supposed to mix it. I just needed the vials. I can't believe this. Now I can't use it 'cause I don't know what's in it."

Anja: [*Why is she so upset? What is she talking about?*] "What do you mean? I listed everything on the label." [*She doesn't trust me.*]

Nurse: "It's against the law for me to inject this into a patient unless I've mixed it myself. How do I know you didn't make a mistake? I'm not going to lose my license over this."

Anja: [*Lose your license over what? I did this right!*] "Sorry. I always mix it for Pediatrics."

Nurse: "That's because Pediatrics is lazy; they don't care. They can lose their licenses if they want to."

Anja: [*Why did I go to school for years only to not be trusted as a professional?*] "Sorry, I didn't know it was against the law. I've been mixing them like this for years and I did put everything in that was on the label. But I'll bring it back and get you a couple of vials and you can do it." [*No more favors for her after this.*]

Nurse: "No, forget it."

Anja: "No, I don't mind."

Nurse: "No, I'll use it; it's just that I told your pharmacy director last week that I didn't want any pre-mixed brought up here."

Anja: [*He could have told me.*] "Sorry, I didn't know 'cause he didn't tell me. Then again, he hardly ever tells me anything."

Case Commentary

What Happened?

Anja worked diligently to make up this medication order correctly and to deliver it in a reasonable amount of time. In return for this effort, she ended up feeling very much like she was slapped in the face. It seems like the nurse doesn't even realize how insulted Anja felt and that is not surprising considering Anja didn't really let her know. Anja is a real accommodator, much too willing to yield easily. She hid the fact that she was very upset.

How Did Unspoken Thoughts and Assumptions Affect the Interaction?

At first Anja is confused about why there is a problem, but she never states this puzzlement aloud. As soon as she understands the nurse's complaint she feels hurt because she feels that she is not trusted. Anja is filling her mind up with reasons that she is trustworthy (her schooling, etc.) without stepping back to ask herself why she needs excessive justifications. By the end of the conversation, she is so hurt that she has reacted with resentful feelings toward both the nurse and her boss. It seems more likely that she is really angry about not standing up for herself.

How Did the Communication Strategies Affect the Outcome?

Anja is very self-deprecating. Notice how many sentences she begins with the word "sorry." The nurse speaks in a very extreme manner, yet Anja never addresses her alarm (e.g., "How do I know you didn't make a mistake?"). Anja is the model doormat, trying to protect peace and harmony at the expense of what she knows is right. From the very start when the nurse said: "What's this?" Anja should have been much more direct and said, "It's the Rocephin you ordered. I gather from your tone that there might be a problem?" Anja needed to show her ability to engage as an equal partner right from the very beginning. Anja also needed to resist the temptation to shift the blame onto her boss at the end. When feeling uncomfortable, it is always too easy to put the spotlight on someone who isn't around.

How Could This Have Been Handled Differently?

Anja needed to bring out her feelings of being mistrusted. She needed to say: "I can see that you're shocked that this is premixed, and although I am sure you did not intend to imply that I'm incompetent, when you say things like, 'I don't know what's in it,' I feel mistrusted. I also feel like you haven't enough confidence in my schooling and professionalism," . . . or, "Frankly, I'm a little shocked by your statement about it being against the law; I've never heard that before and I'd like to talk to my boss about it because it has implications for a different delivery system for many units. For now, I can give you this premixed vial with my assurance, or I can go get you some new vials. Either way I guess we need to talk again about this issue. . . ." Anja needs to show that she is willing to solve the problem with long-term solutions rather that becoming paralyzed and capitulating in the moment.

Chapter 8

The Consequences of Choosing
New Communication Options

After reviewing the preceding cases, the careful reader may be a bit alarmed. Is it expected or even desired that pharmacists use different interpersonal strategies each and every time they talk with a patient or co-worker? Rest assured that the author does not advocate repeating word for word all the suggestions given under the "How else could this have been handled?" sections. These suggestions were not given as a definitive list of things to say or not say. In fact, beginning with just one new communication strategy (e.g., empathic listening) and employing it consistently can create significant changes in communication. There is room for expanding on the insights provided and it is expected that individuals will adapt the ideas to their own speaking style. All people would benefit from adding to their repertoire of behavioral options, though there may be great resistance to doing so because change of this type is not easy, and it often feels unnatural and awkward.

THE DEVELOPMENTAL STAGES
OF INTERPERSONAL SKILLS IMPROVEMENT

As a facilitator of interpersonal skills training workshops, the author makes frequent suggestions to participants about how else they could have handled a particular situation. A very common response to these ideas is: "But I couldn't say that 'cause it doesn't sound like me!" This may be so, but it also may be that we need to constantly evolve our voice to meet new, present and future demands. It seems that just when we master the skills of being an outstanding pharmacy student we are thrust into being an entry-level pharmacist. When the skills of being a staff pharmacist feel automatic and "mastered," someone offers us a promotion to supervisor (and so on).

Change in interpersonal skills does not happen overnight; it is a developmental, ongoing process. Let's look at some hypothetical stages along the way from naiveté to skilled competence. A specific interpersonal situation may be useful in illustrating this process, and the dreaded dilemma of asking for a raise should be of interest to most people (Deetz and Stevenson, 1986).

Individuals in stage one of interpersonal skills development will believe that all bosses are basically alike and they formulate little useful information beyond this conclusion. They will march into a session with the boss and ask for the money and hope it goes well. If it doesn't go well, they will probably decide: "I knew he didn't like me." The subtleties of the boss's perspective are likely to be missed.

In stage two of interpersonal skills development, the individual can perceive that not all bosses are alike. Some supervisors have worked their way up through the trenches and others have been "sponsored" by rich relatives who own the drugstore. Still, knowing this type of information is confusing with regard to what might be relevant and irrelevant and what should be "used" or "not used" in formulating a strategy.

When people are operating in stage three of interpersonal skills development, they can read other's reactions more sensitively. They know when to back off because they may have applied too much pressure. These individuals have more ideas about how to handle the situation and they recognize that they are not always capable of following through. If they fail to get the raise, they are likely to see it as a situation where they needed additional skills, rather than projecting the blame onto an uncaring, unresponsive, "big bad boss."

Those individuals in the fourth level of skills development have some general strategies that they can employ in a number of situations. They may believe that emotional appeals reap rewards and therefore they ask for the boss's sympathy with regard to supporting five hungry children on only a cost-of-living adjustment. They see themselves as taking a gamble, their strategy may "work" or it may "backfire," but it's worth a try.

In the final stage of interpersonal skills development, people are unwilling to achieve individual gain at the cost of mutual respect. They are willing to collaborate and the message given the boss will be adaptive. They will probably acknowledge past work accomplishments, weaknesses, and areas for improvement in present work practices and plans for work in the future. They will raise only relevant truths in the quest for a raise, all the while being sensitive to the larger system of constraints' impacting on the boss's behavior. If they have some assumptions about the forces operating on the boss's behavior they will find an effective way to bring them into the discussion without evaluating, raising voices, pulling power plays, or any other behavior that is ultimately counterproductive, no matter how good it may feel at the moment (Deetz and Stevenson, 1986).

WHAT DOES THE INTERNAL UNSPOKEN DIALOGUE OF THE CASE STUDIES REVEAL?

By analyzing the thinking patterns in the internal dialogue, some predictable patterns are discernable. The pharmacists generally hold the other party in the case to be more responsible for negative outcomes than positive ones. If the nurse remembers to call first before arriving at the pharmacy to pick up a medication, it is because she is reasonably considerate. If she does not call it is because she is stupid and self-centered. Of course, when it comes to relations between the health care team, it is obviously a greater sin to be perceived as lazy rather than merely incompetent. It is worse to be perceived as pulling rank and being on a power trip rather than merely trying to save face. The fundamental error that people created in their internal dialogue can be summed up as follows: "Jane and John Doe were perfectly free to act as they wished but they *chose* to be unreasonable because that is the type of people they are." Basically we hold other people more responsible for their behavior than we think we are for our own behavior. In brief, they cause their own problems and we excuse ours (Griffin, 1991).

Few people are as good or as bad as we want to believe. In every major criminal court case many jurors are excused for bias, but the rest of us continue to pass judgement every day in the court of interpersonal injustice! For example, you might be told, "You know, you really blew it big time when you asked the boss for time off. First you have to see if he's in a good mood, butter him up and then. . . ." We draw inferences about other's behavior by projecting our own habits and styles onto theirs as a kind of measuring yardstick. This process happens in steps. First we perceive ("I saw you behave rudely to that last customer"), then we attribute intent ("You meant to be abrupt"), and lastly we infer disposition ("You're not fit to work with the public"). This three-step process (see Griffin, 1991) plays out in milliseconds in our minds and faster than we can become conscious of it we have passed judgement and issued our reactive sentence (double entendré intended).

The unspoken dialogue in many of the cases also reveals the "catastrophic" response of feeling totally incompetent because of a minor interpersonal incident. An absence of self-coaching behavior is noticeable. There is a difference between *knowing you should* say or not say something and *knowing how* to make that communicative choice. Instead we play out our familiar patterns and "social recipes" for responding to interpersonal behavior (Deetz and Stevenson, 1986). So many of the cases have a back and forth, "vicious cycle" quality and yet without knowing how to stop it, we cannot see that doing more of the same behavior is simply not getting us anywhere.

WHY DO CUSTOMERS AND CO-WORKERS GET EMOTIONALLY UPSET?

When patients or co-workers get upset, it is often because they are tired, scared, confused, overwhelmed, trying to save face, embarrassed, dealing with unknowns, in a hurry, or were treated poorly in the past. Most of these reasons are beyond the control of the health care provider. On the other hand, some emotional upsets are entirely avoidable. Examples of these situations include: when a promise wasn't fulfilled; having to repeat themselves because of poor listening; being told, "You have no business being upset, other customers have it worse than you"; or receiving a flip reply to a sincere question (Morgan, 1989). It is important for the health care provider to determine whether the person is upset for avoidable or unavoidable reasons. Either way, the preceding cases have made clear that an automatic robotic response of "sorry" is not a psychologically satisfying response. Empathic reflection is usually the best response to the unavoidable upsets, but in the case of the avoidable problems, the service provider should first *thank the customer for raising the problem*, and tell them, "That's not the kind of service we want to provide, so I really wish that had not happened to you." Follow up with collaborative problem-solving strategies to solve the situation in such a way that it is fully resolved (Martin, 1989).

Above all else, avoid making the situation worse by saying things like: "Sorry I didn't call you about this, I got stuck in a meeting"; "I don't understand why the doctor didn't explain this to you"; "My boss is in a meeting, why don't you call back in a while?"; "I hope this will do the trick"; "We have had a lot of problems with our suppliers, maybe I can try to find out if your medication will come in soon." We all have it in us to drive our customers and co-workers even crazier! Even statements that are very well-meaning can be problematic when they contain words like hope, try, and maybe. In their upset state, ambiguous terms such as "maybe" feel like salt in the wound to the patient already in psychic pain. The author is struck by the number of "dealing with difficult people" seminars there are being offered in the country today (and she offers many of them). When health care providers sign up for these seminars they are often expecting to learn who to watch out for and who to avoid. Of course, the real truth of the matter is that "We have met the difficult person and *they is us!*"

WHY IS IT SO EASY TO PASS ALONG NEGATIVE BEHAVIOR?

We live in a world that tolerates and sometimes encourages interpersonal violence (anyone who has driven in urban traffic in a major northeast city can easily verify this). Subsequently, many of us are "conditioned" to think or feel that we won't get what we want or think we need unless we exert force. "No one listens until you yell" is an operating premise for a significant percentage of our population. Some people give the impression that they are not happy unless they are mad! Recently in an interpersonal skills for pharmacy practice course, a young man came in and began boasting loudly to his fellow classmates about how the college registrar had messed up his registration, and he yelled at her and belittled her until she fixed it right away. The instructor, who couldn't help overhearing the conversation, turned to the young man and said, "And how is that situation different from one in which you have a belligerent customer screaming in your face, 'Don't tell me I can't have another refill; I want it now!'?" The student was stunned to realize that he had passed on the type of everyday abuse that made his job in the pharmacy so stressful.

Stopping the everyday abuse cycle does not mean that pharmacists should become passive, smile all the time, and continuously say "Yes sir" or "Yes ma'am." This text is not advocating that pharmacists unilaterally disarm all their defenses and coping strategies until they feel like sitting ducks unprepared to protect themselves. In fact, in rereading the cases it can be noted that the alternatives for communication described in the "How could this have been handled differently?" sections do not consist of "overly polite" or "nice" behaviors. There is an implicit premise in the minds of participants in interpersonal skills workshops that college professors and consultants have never dealt with John and Jane Q. Public. As any teacher who has ever disagreed with a student over a grade can tell you, we deal with plenty of upset people in our professional practice.

At the extreme, there is behavior designed to "teach the patient a lesson." Pharmacists have told the author stories of adding an extra ten dollars onto an Rx price out of sheer frustration and revenge. Others have admitted to making rude customers wait much longer as a way of retaliating. One pharmacist in a workshop shared his "secret strategy" for getting rid of pests on the phone. Instead of hanging up on someone who is problematic while they are dishing out their complaints, he waits until he is talking and then clicks down the receiver mid-sentence. He gloated to our workshop group: "When you hang up on yourself they never think you did it; they always think they got disconnected. It works every time! When they call back, I have the tech answer and give them a story." The evidence of burnout in pharmacy customer service is very profound indeed!

Still there is this persistent concern that "nice guys (or gals) finish last." We are afraid not to participate in our world aggressively enough, and subsequently, we feel stuck in patterns of relating we don't like. We often feel that it is not safe for us to change our behavior until "they" (the boss, the customer, the spouse, the government, etc.) change their behavior first. It seems that the implicit unconscious assumption here is that others will continue to behave the same way regardless of our behavior. We see our options in a polarized fashion: either protect ourselves or leave ourselves wide open to attack in a dangerous world. We act as if we have absolutely no influence on the dynamics of the interactions that make up our lives. Rarely do we realize that others are feeling trapped in similar ways and would welcome the modeling of different behavior (Lewis, 1992).

SO WHAT DOES THE UPSET CUSTOMER OR CO-WORKER WANT FROM US?

When upset over how a situation has turned out, the biggest fear people have is that they will have to go through this all over again the next time they deal with you or your organization. The most bitter and burnt out among us want punishment of a guilty party, while most people will be appeased with being treated with respect, taken seriously, given restitution, or offered emotional comfort in a timely manner (Morgan, 1989). To handle an upset person it is crucial to solve the problem without blaming yourself ("I can't believe I forgot!") or them ("Like you're perfect yourself, buddy!"). It is the *relationship* that matters not who is *right* and who is *wrong*. Things are seldom as black and white as "victim" and "victimizer"-type thinking would suggest. When we look at communication as a transactional system, it makes it easier for each person to own their piece of the problem. The "He started it" defense is awfully weak when it is obvious that the reaction is generally a case of "I'll meet that insult and injury and raise the ante." Vicious cycles don't usually have clear-cut beginnings and endings.

WHY DO WE HAVE TO THINK ABOUT
COMMUNICATION SKILLS SO CONSCIOUSLY?

As this book is being written, we are living in an age of fierce competition in health care. Total quality management seminars are being provided to health care professionals in hospitals, health maintenance organizations, and retail practice all over the country. Excellence in customer service makes good economic sense and makes the job less stressful. Communication competence is a transferable skill which improves our chances of promotion and the likelihood that we can succeed in new positions in any organization. Conversely, failure to communicate well is not something we can hide from the outside world. In fact, research in customer service indicates that if one customer feels that he was treated poorly he will tell eleven people about it. Those eleven people will each tell five people so that a total of 65 people will have heard that your organization is not providing quality service (Morgan, 1989).

RECOGNIZING BURNOUT
IN "PEOPLE SKILLS"-ORIENTED JOBS

Most pharmacists resent the image that all they do is count pills and type labels. Still, while conducting an interpersonal skills workshop, a pharmacist told the author, "I hate all these new mandatory counseling laws because I hate talking to people! Leave me alone and let me count my pills and type labels; I prefer it over talking to customers." Obviously, this pharmacist is not exactly set up for success. He would rather work with things than people, he likes order and predictable events, and subsequently, in an era of great change in pharmacy practice, he feels depressed, angry, and stuck in his job. If he doesn't start asking himself "What else could I have said or done to help that person?" he is on a collision course with total burnout. So many of the cases we have analyzed feature people who have burnt out and they may or may not realize it consciously.

Granted, the pharmacist mentioned above is an extreme case that most pharmacists would not identify with. So what are some of the more typical signs of burnout in people-oriented jobs? If you find yourself saying out loud or to yourself, "I don't get paid enough to take this garbage," "No one appreciates me," "They always . . . ," "They never . . . ," "Who is he to talk to me like that?", you are not exercising your communication options effectively. To verify your self-diagnosis, examine your behavior after you go home from work. Do you abuse the "Plug-in drug"? Are you dependent on too much caffeine? Do you feel drained or apathetic? Are you having sleeping or eating disturbances? Is decreased concentration and a short fuse a problem? And as a final test, are you suspicious of people who seem up, joyful, and love their jobs and life in general (Martin, 1989)?

If these signs of burnout are hauntingly familiar, it would be beneficial to look back over some of the case studies again. Pick out the scenarios that most often parallel situations in which you find yourself. Concentrate on the section: "How could this have been handled differently?" The discussions under these headings are only an initial examination of options for coping with challenging situations. The key is often finding ways to increase our collaborative communication strategies.

PAYING CAREFUL ATTENTION TO OUR COMMUNICATION CHOICES

The famous linguists Sapir and Whorf developed a theory that states that the language we use shapes our perceptions of the reality of the world around us (DeVito, 1989). If this is true, learning new language use habits may help us to reframe our lives and see new and increased options for behavior. Although it may seem like a simple and insignificant difference, let's look at some ways to reframe language so that it is more positive. Instead of saying, "You can't have this today," why not say, "You can have this by tomorrow morning." Don't say "I'll try to call your doctor," say, "I will call your doctor's office"! Instead of the robotic "Phone number, please?" which often provokes, "You've got it; why do I get asked every time?" give the reason right up front, "So that I can verify your records may I ask you your phone number again?" Paying attention to the subtleties of language use pays off in positive reactions from the people we deal with.

The value of listening and careful responding was brought home to the author in a humorous way on a recent visit to her neighborhood pharmacy to purchase a very expensive round of antibiotics for a persistent ear infection. The pharmacists on duty were all former students of the author and as usual when they saw her approach, the bunch began to tease: "I'm not talking to you. It will just end up in your book or you'll tell the story at a seminar." A new tech had just come on duty so they brought her out to deal with this "difficult" customer. I handed over my Rx forms and she asked, "Did they tell you at the hospital about this medication?" (a closed, leading question), to which I said, "Sounds like you're worried that I might be upset when I find out how expensive it is." She then said, "Yeah, *exactly!* The last five people took a nutty on me when I told them; you wouldn't believe how some people can be!" My former students who were eavesdropping looked at me and smiled and I thought of all the times we had debated whether or not reflective empathic listening works. Clearly it helped the pharmacy tech to feel that someone did understand.

Not everyone with whom you exercise your best people skills will respond in kind. If an interaction with a co-worker or customer goes badly, it is important to review it rather than try to forget it. What could you have done to avoid contributing to a vicious cycle? What did you say that you don't want to say again? What can you learn from this? It is important not to internalize the other person's reactive anger. And it is very important not to vent your frustration or anger on a co-worker afterwards (Morgan, 1989). This process is discouraging, sends a negative message, and introduces more burnout and stress into the workplace atmosphere. So often when venting with a co-worker after an incident we send the message, "I did everything humanly possible to deal with that idiot but he was impossible to deal with!" Really? Everything possible in all of the infinite universe? These types of statements do not invite feedback from our co-workers, who may indeed have an idea or two about another way to handle such a situation.

IF WE FAIL TO CHANGE
OUR AUTOMATIC COMMUNICATION HABITS,
WHAT RESULTS CAN WE EXPECT?

The key issue throughout the cases in the text is one of learning to take conscious action rather than have an unreflective reaction. For example, if in our perception someone is "giving us a hard time," we usually try to strengthen our counterarguments against their arguments and, without realizing it, add more volume, speed, and force to our speech. Raising voices into a shouting match is not an elegant solution to an interpersonal problem.

By being reactive, we enact self-fulfilling prophecies. If we think of the unit nurses as only being capable of a few typical reactions to drug delivery problems, we will subconsciously find a way to provoke these behaviors from them. Falling into these patterns does not stimulate our critical thinking and multiple perspective-taking skills. Retail pharmacists often have a system for editorializing on the patient's profiles. P.I.A., as an acronym for "pain in the ass," is the system most often reported to be used. Imagine you are counseling an elderly woman and things seem to be going just fine. You then pull up her profile and notice a very large P.I.A. with other illustrative comments on the screen. It will be difficult to finish your counseling session in the same state of mind that you started it and if she picks up on your tension, she will react to it. If she seems the slightest bit ornery you can then blame her for "starting something."

All of us who have been socialized in American culture have feelings of needing to cover inadequacies rather than enlisting help. The American way is so competitive it even shows up in our northeast urban driving habits. The unwritten rules of the road go like this, "When you want to change lanes, (1) Don't signal; (2) Get the nose of your car in front of the person you are cutting off; (3) Don't look at the other human being, never make eye contact! Keep face steely, determined, and straight ahead in the desired path." Imagine the shock on people's faces if you signalled, made direct eye contact, waved and gestured, mouthing the words to indicate you are asking to cut in, and then waved to say thanks. This *rare* behavior produces enough shock value in the other driver that they inevitably let you pass while they are feeling totally stunned. This is completely analogous to interpersonal behavior. Though you may still be doubtful, if you try some of the other strategies suggested in the "How could this have been handled differently?" sections, you may experience some pleasant surprises.

Thinking back over the cases you have read, you will notice that the internal dialogue does not keep people focused on how they are contributing to the interpersonal process. This automatic process of diagnosing the other but not ourselves keeps us stuck in a number of ways. Our thinking is very much like the simple house thermostat. The thermostat never asks itself if it is set on an effective setting given the realities of what season it is, or whether it should be doing it's part to conserve electricity, etc. Like that automatic thermostat, we simply promulgate our own status quo (Argyris, 1990). Similarly, simply knowing your Myers Briggs personality type doesn't give you the communication skills you need to make radical changes in your life. We need new ways to "learn how to learn" from our own behavior. If you go home and complain to your family and friends,"You wouldn't believe the jerks I had to work with today," you are not inviting them to help you reflect on how you might have handled things in other ways than you did.

If we fail to try something different we will end up exhausted, brittle, powerless, and burnt out. We need to accept that we all have a "King Lear" level of self-blindness, and that we are blind to the fact that we cannot self-diagnose ourselves instantly, easily, or accurately. Only when we see this does life get less punishing and more exciting and fascinating.

WHAT WOULD OUR COMMUNICATION CHOICES LOOK LIKE IF WE MADE THEM DIFFERENTLY?

As has been the approach of this book throughout, let's look at an example of a "traditional" way of handling a tough interpersonal situation versus a different way of approaching the same problem.

The process of firing a problematic employee usually plays out as follows: (1) Build up evidence so that it looks like a sure case of incompetence or negligence and so on; (2) Tell the worker that he or she is a perfectly good person but that it is a question of "fit" with the organization; (3) Offer a good financial separation package; (4) Offer to lie to references for future jobs (Argyris, 1990).

A different way of handling the situation would be to say to the employee, "At the moment we believe that you are having difficulty performing this job because of our observations of.... We are telling you early because we want to check our perceptions to see if we are right or wrong about this. Maybe we don't have a complete picture of your work so we would like to design a series of tests *with you* that we both could agree would confirm or disconfirm our current conclusions." Many will react: "That sounds awfully inhumane! Giving the employees enough rope to hang themselves?" True, it would be cruel if the manager has decided in advance that the employee will fail. If this is the case, the self-fulfilling prophesy dynamic will come into play in an unfortunate way. But if the manager is open and *co-designs* a series of tests that the employee agrees is fair, she has actually been much more humane than if she had silently stockpiled ammunition from a biased viewpoint. If after going through this process the decision to let the employee go is confirmed, there is a greater likelihood that this individual will not go forth and gossip negatively about how he or she was treated.

Although the case of having to fire someone is an extreme example, it can be seen that acting in a different way from what we usually see modeled in the world can bring rich rewards. Some solutions are more psychologically satisfying than others no matter what the actual outcome is in terms of money or material goods. "Psychic income" is a concept that is useful as we assess the quality of our lives. For instance, if under the new mandatory counseling laws, pharmacists must counsel but may not always get reimbursed, how will they maintain morale? Becoming more conscious of unconscious, automatic behaviors and attitudes takes effort and will feel awkward at first. New kinds of self and other analysis are threatening, but true insight brings tremendous relief.

CONCLUDING THOUGHTS

It is the act of an ill-instructed man to blame others for his own bad condition; it is the act of one who has begun to be instructed to lay the blame on himself, and of one whose instruction has been completed, neither to blame another, nor himself.

–Epictetus

When significant new insights about effective interpersonal skills are achieved, it is tempting to look back at situations from the past and feel bad that "If we only knew then what we know now." Many workplace relationships gone bad end in mutual recrimination, hurt innocent parties along the way, and make for a negative work environment. It is hard to stop our personal contributions to interpersonal pollution, let alone clean up after a human relations toxic spill. Each of us carries the burden of past and present skills deficits and each of us must contribute to a vision of a peopled environment that has a sustainable future. Even a casual reading of a daily newspaper indicates that the world's supply of positive behavior is in serious jeopardy!

There will be internal and external pressures to backslide from newly acquired skills development. Long-established patterns of behavior are hard to break. Our motivation to change diminishes if we play the comparison game ("My boss doesn't bother to counsel patients; why should I?"). Peers may apply pressure ("Going out of your way for the customers makes the rest of us look bad. Can you ease up a bit?"). Still, commitment to your own and other's development means not seeing people as means to an end (Nelson-Jones, 1990).

Having hurtful interactions and not being able to set appropriate limits is exhausting. It is important to contract with yourself to set a goal of personal excellence. There are a number of ways to help yourself to achieve this level of practice. Tell your co-workers about your goals by introducing them one step at a time (e.g., "I'm trying to stop interrupting so much; can you tell me when you hear me cutting you off?"). Go to training seminars that focus on behavioral skills in addition to clinically based updates. Start a support group of pharmacists with similar interests who can commit to meet on a realistic schedule of frequency. Read relevant articles in pharmacy-, management-, and psychology-oriented journals and periodicals. Self-monitor your talking patterns. Remember the study cited in the opening chapter that indicated that people remember ninety percent of what they themselves say. In light of this research, always remember *to talk with* your patients and co-workers instead of simply *talking at* them.

Perhaps most importantly, try your hand at writing up your own case study. The act of capturing what you said versus what you did not say provides significant insights. By reflecting on your own communication in your own case, you should be able to transfer the learning directly to your on-the-job behavior. By maintaining a skills orientation, we remove the temptation to simply write off every positive experience with people as "luck" and every negative experience as the result of someone else's "bad mood." Although it is clear that a seminar with the title "Everyday Communication Skills" would draw fewer participants than a workshop on "Crisis Management Strategies," it is important to see that the practice of all of our people skills has a common core that can and should be put to the test continuously.

Maybe the day is coming when pharmacists will be as highly rewarded for their human relations skills as they are for filling a large number of scripts per day. Pharmacists must constantly review whether or not their personal practice skills are hurtful or helpful. To improve the professional practice of pharmacy, we must nurture the communication competencies of today's and tomorrow's pharmacists.

References

Adler, R. and Rodman, C. 1982. *Understanding Human Communication*. New York: Holt, Rhinehart and Winston.

Anastasi, T. 1982. *Listen! Techniques for Improving Communication*. Boston: C.B.I. Publishing.

Argyris, C. 1990. *Overcoming Organizational Defenses*. Needham, MA: Allyn and Bacon.

Arnold, E. and McClure, L. 1989. *Communication Training and Development*. New York: Harper and Row.

Bolton, R. 1979. *People Skills*. New York: Simon and Schuster.

Dance, F. and Larson, C. 1972. *Speech Communication: Concepts and Behavior*. New York: Holt, Rhinehart and Winston.

Deetz, S. and Stevenson, S. 1986. *Managing Interpersonal Communication*. New York: Harper and Row.

DeVito, J. 1989. *The Interpersonal Communication Book* (5th Ed.). New York: Harper and Row.

Gardner, M., Boyce, R., and Herrier, R. 1991. *Pharmacist-Patient Consultation Program*. New York: Pfizer Inc. Training Program.

Glasser, S. 1983. "Communication Instruction: A Behavioral Competency Approach." *Communication Education*, Vol. 32, pp. 221-225.

Griffin, E. 1991. *A First Look at Communication Theory*. New York: McGraw-Hill.

Habel, D. 1991. "Obstacles to Excellence: Factors Leading to an Exaggerated Sense of Communication Proficiency." Presented to the Eastern Communication Association, Pittsburgh, PA.

Johnson, D. 1986. *Reaching Out* (3rd Ed.). Englewood Cliffs, NJ: Prentice Hall.

Kennedy, E. 1977. *On Becoming a Counselor*. New York: The Seabury Press.

Lewis, S. 1992. Personal Communication. Cambridge, MA.

Lynch, J. 1985. *The Language of the Heart: The Body's Response to Human Dialogue*. New York: Basic Books.

Martin, W. 1989. *Quality Customer Service.* Los Altos, CA: Crisp Publications.

Meldrum, H. 1986. "Communication Options." Somerville, MA: Communication Counseling Associates.

Meldrum, H. 1990. "Communicating with the Mentally Ill." Somerville, MA: Communication Counseling Associates.

Meldrum, H. and Rando, W. 1987. "Using Self-Authored Case Studies to Reduce Defensiveness and Increase Interpersonal Awareness." Conference on Therapeutic Communication, Chicago.

Morgan, R. 1989. *Calming Upset Customers.* Los Altos, CA: Crisp Publications.

Nelson-Jones, R. 1990. *Human Relationships, A Skills Approach.* Belmont, CA: Wadsworth.

Tannen, D. 1986. *That's Not What I Meant!* New York: Ballantine Books.

Tindall, W., Beardsley, R. and Kimberlin, C. 1989. *Communication Skills in Pharmacy Practice* (2nd Ed.). Philadelphia: Lea and Ferbiger.

Tuttle, G. 1985. *Introduction to Speech Communication* (2nd Ed.). Prospect Heights, IL: Waveland Press.

Index